W9-ATO-791

How to
GROW
your
family

How to
GROW
your
family

From pregnancy
to new parents –
one meal at a time

Adam Shaw

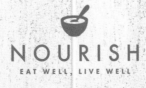

NOURISH

EAT WELL, LIVE WELL

This book is dedicated first of all to my amazing wife Anni. You not only inspired me to start At Dad's Table but gave me all the encouragement to try and make something of it. I love you and thank you. And thank you for keeping the boys occupied while I was cooking and writing! To my wonderful two boys, Basti and Benji. I'm hoping this will help explain a bit more what Daddy's job is now! ("Why does Daddy keep taking a picture of my dinner by the window?") Thank you for being my tasters-in-chiefs and for being brutally, brutally honest when you didn't like a dish.

This book is also dedicated to everyone who follows me on At Dad's Table, whether you've been there from the start or just come on board. Thank you for your kind messages, your time but, most importantly, thank you for your support as without you this book would never have come about! I really hope you enjoy the recipes. Love, Adam

How to Grow Your Family
Adam Shaw

First published in the UK and USA in 2022 by Nourish, an imprint of Watkins Media Limited Unit 11, Shepperton House, 83–93 Shepperton Road London N1 3DF enquiries@nourishbooks.com

Copyright © Watkins Media Limited 2022
Text and photography copyright © Adam Shaw 2022
Artwork copyright © Watkins Media Limited 2022

The right of Adam Shaw to be identified as the Author of this text has been asserted in accordance with the Copyright, Designs and Patents Act of 1988.

All rights reserved. No part of this book may be reproduced in any form or by any electronic or mechanical means, including information storage and retrieval systems, without permission in writing from the publisher, except by a reviewer who may quote brief passages in a review.

Commissioning Editor: Ella Chappell
Copy Editor: Sophie Elletson
Proofreader: Nicole Bator
Nutritionist: Dr Michelle Braude
Head of Design: Karen Smith
Designer: Alice Claire Coleman
Production: Uzma Taj
Food photography: Adam Shaw (@At_Dads_Table)
Logo design: Matt Hunt @hellomatt
Family Photography: Emily Butters Photography
@emilybuttersphotography

A CIP record for this book is available from the British Library

ISBN: 978-1-84899-396-9 (Hardback)
ISBN: 978-1-84899-397-6 (eBook)

10 9 8 7 6 5 4 3 2 1

Typeset in Pulpo and Futura
Printed in Bosnia and Herzegovina

Publisher's note
While every care has been taken in compiling the recipes for this book, Watkins Media Limited, or any other persons who have been involved in working on this publication, cannot accept responsibility for any errors or omissions, inadvertent or not, that may be found in the recipes or text, nor for any problems that may arise as a result of preparing one of these recipes. If you are pregnant or breastfeeding or have any special dietary requirements or medical conditions, it is advisable to consult a medical professional before following any of the recipes contained in this book.

Notes on the recipes
Unless otherwise stated:
Use medium fruit and vegetables
Use medium (US large) organic or free-range eggs
Use fresh herbs, spices and chillies
Use granulated sugar (Americans can use ordinary granulated sugar when caster sugar is specified)
Do not mix metric, imperial and US cup measurements:
1 tsp = 5ml 1 tbsp = 15ml 1 cup = 240ml

nourishbooks.com

Contents

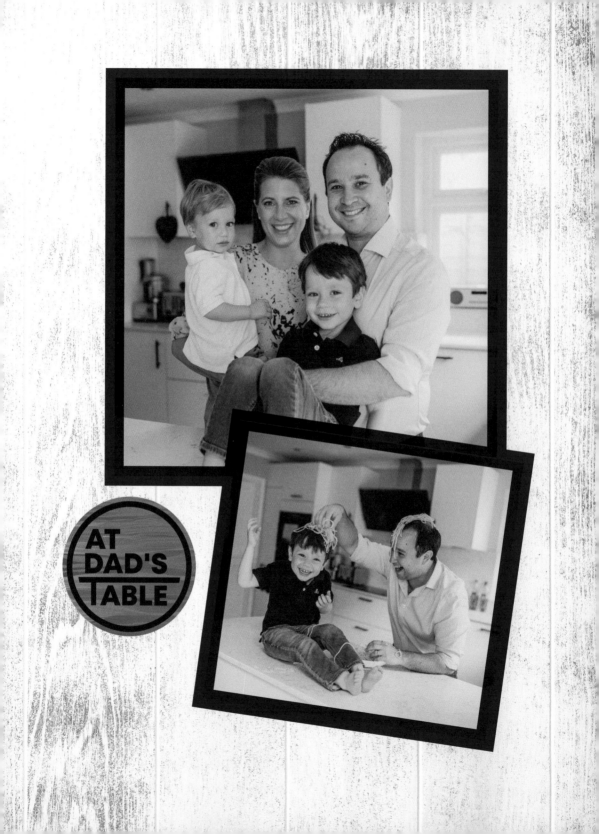

AT
DAD'S
TABLE

Introduction

Welcome to How to Grow Your Family! I'm Adam, a proud husband and father to two young boys (Basti and Benji) born in 2017 and 2020. I'm also a trained chef and regularly post on Instagram at @At_Dads_Table, where I've built up a community of thousands of foodies and parents around the world.

My story

This book really came about through love. A few years ago, I fulfilled a long-held ambition of mine and trained after work at the prestigious Leiths School of Food and Wine in London. A few months later when my wife Anni became pregnant for the first time I was really looking forward to putting my new skills to use and cooking lots of healthy and delicious food for her and our unborn baby. However, after doing some research I became disheartened with the available guidance for eating in pregnancy as it seemed to focus on what you can't eat, rather than what you can. The whole issue of food in pregnancy was framed in this rather pessimistic narrative instead of what food should be: **a way to make yourself feel good**. It was as if overnight Anni was expected to go from someone who loved eating lots of varied foods to someone who should now restrict and deny herself.

So, I decided to design my own recipes to accompany my wife's pregnancy and At Dad's Table was born. I focused on all the wonderful foods she could eat at that special time – food that was not only good for her, but made her feel good too. I also tailored different recipes to different trimesters when the nutritional requirements change slightly and mum-to-be can experience changes in not only how she feels but what she wants to eat.

When our first child Sebastian was born, we both found ourselves sledgehammer-hit in the face by how life changed. My wife was home alone caring for our newborn while I was working, commuting and out of the house for 12 hours a day. There just wasn't enough time in the day for either of us to get everything done. Amongst the never-ending to-do list, I didn't want to sacrifice eating well, so I designed quick, high-energy meals for both of us that were also suitable for batch-cooking and were therefore timesaving. With me out of the house all day and Anni spending all her time with Basti, food she could prepare and eat with one hand was also crucial!

When Basti turned six months, we started to wean him and after a few weeks of vegetable purées I began to include him in what Anni and I ate each day (although a few things obviously needed to be adapted slightly). I think it's really important that as soon as baby has tried some first foods and been exposed to allergens that they experience as many different tastes and flavours as possible. Plus, from a time-saving perspective, it made sense to just make one meal for the whole family. A few months later my wife became pregnant with our second son Benji and we started the whole process from scratch again!

As a partner I've found that cooking for my pregnant wife and then my family has helped me to stay involved at a time when, as a working parent, I was missing seeing my family change and a lot of the pressure seemed to be unfairly on the new mum.

Through @At_Dads_Table I've helped thousands of people around the world feel positive about eating well during these crazy, exhausting years and I love the community I've built up online. What with all of life's pressures I am a firm believer in cooking one dish for whoever is sharing your table. At the time of writing, sharing mine is my wonderful wife, a kind, absolute rocket of a threenager and an inquisitive, curious one-year old. These recipes have really helped me to grow my family and I hope they do the same for you.

Love, Adam

Breaking down each chapter

The six chapters in this book cover the journey from early pregnancy all the way through to parenthood, weaning and baby-friendly family recipes. Chapters 1 to 3 cover the carb-craving fog of the first trimester, the eat-the-rainbow second trimester and the energy-loading third trimester. Each recipe is designed to make mum-to-be (and whoever is eating with her) feel good. Chapter 4 details energy-boosting meals for tired new parents as well as one-handed snacks and light dishes for when you're home alone with a newborn you can't quite put down! Chapter 5 explains how to start weaning at six months and features finger foods everyone will enjoy. Chapter 6 finishes with recipes for the whole family, be it hangry parent, toddler or baby.

Each chapter provides an overview of the importance of different foods at different points of the journey and then around 20 recipes (split into brunch, main meals, snacks and something sweet). There are also spotlight sections in each chapter that take one relevant area (getting more veg into meals, batch-cooking, one-handed dips) and go into greater detail.

I'm a working dad of two and I know that time is precious, so most recipes are on the table in around 30 minutes. Alternatives, including plant-based and gluten-free options, are provided, and at the end of the book you'll find a handy list of all ingredients used and their nutritional contents. This way you'll know exactly how each ingredient can combine to give you a plate of food full of the nutrients you need. Each recipe also tells you if it's suitable for batch-cooking and if it's baby- and family-friendly.

While eating well during pregnancy is particularly important, it's worth stating that the recipes in no way replace any vitamins and supplements that mum-to-be is taking. No recipe should be followed if it is in direct conflict with any advice a medical professional has recommended personally.

Equipment

I cook in quite a basic home kitchen, and I want all of my recipes to be accessible to everyone. Beyond the essentials, the items I couldn't live without are a stick blender for making soups and a small hand blender for pesto and purées — both are inexpensive and available from any home-appliance store.

Nutrients for Mum-to-be and Baby

VITAMIN A: Good for your body's immune system, vision, maintaining internal organs and healthy skin. During pregnancy it's important for baby's growth as well as the development of the heart, lungs, eyes, kidneys and bones, and the respiratory, circulatory and central nervous systems.

VITAMINS B1, 2, 3 AND 5: Help break down food and turn it into energy as well as keep skin, eyes and the nervous system healthy. B1 is also important for baby's brain development.

VITAMIN B6: Helps the body to store and use energy from protein and carbohydrate sources. Helps the body form haemoglobin, which carries oxygen around the body in red blood cells. In pregnancy it's important for baby's brain and nervous system development.

VITAMIN B7 (BIOTIN): Helps the body make fatty acids as well as maintain healthy hair and nails.

VITAMIN B9 (FOLATE): Helps the body form red blood cells and reduces the risk of birth defects like spina bifida.

VITAMIN B12: Helps the body make red blood cells and keeps the nervous system healthy. It also helps release energy from food. In pregnancy it helps develop baby's spine and central nervous system.

VITAMIN C: Helps protect cells and keep them healthy as well as maintain healthy skin, blood vessels, bones and cartilage. In pregnancy it helps baby's bone and teeth develop.

VITAMIN D: Helps regulate the amount of calcium in the body which is responsible for keeping teeth, bones and muscles healthy. In pregnancy it helps baby's bones, teeth, heart, kidneys and nervous system develop.

VITAMIN E: Helps maintain healthy skin and eyes and strengthens the immune system.

VITAMIN K: Helps develop and keep bones healthy and helps blood to clot.

CALCIUM: Helps build and develop strong bones and teeth. It also boosts nerve, muscle and heart development, regulates muscle contractions (like your heartbeat) and makes sure blood clots normally.

COPPER: Helps produce red and white blood cells and triggers the release of iron to form haemoglobin, which carries oxygen around the body. Copper also helps form your baby's heart, blood vessels, skeletal and nervous systems.

FIBRE: Essential for maintaining a healthy digestive system.

IRON: Very important in the creation of red blood cells. This is especially true in pregnancy, when mum-to-be is creating more blood to supply oxygen to baby.

MAGNESIUM: Helps turn food into energy and build strong teeth and bones. Regulates insulin and blood sugar levels and builds and repairs tissues.

MANGANESE: Helps the body form connective tissue, bones, blood clotting factors and sex hormones.

OMEGA-3 FATTY ACIDS: Support brain and eye development.

PHOSPHOROUS: Helps build and repair bones and teeth and helps nerves function and muscles contract.

POTASSIUM: Helps control the balance of fluids in the body as well as helps the heart muscle to work properly.

PROTEIN: For building and repairing muscles and bones as well as making hormones and enzymes. Protein is also a source of energy. In pregnancy it ensures the normal growth of tissues and organs, including the brain.

SELENIUM: Essential for thyroid health and a working metabolism.

ZINC: Helps make new cells. Processes protein, carbohydrates and fat in foods.

The recipes in this book should in no way replace any vitamins and supplements that should be taken during pregnancy and beyond.

Source: www.nhs.uk

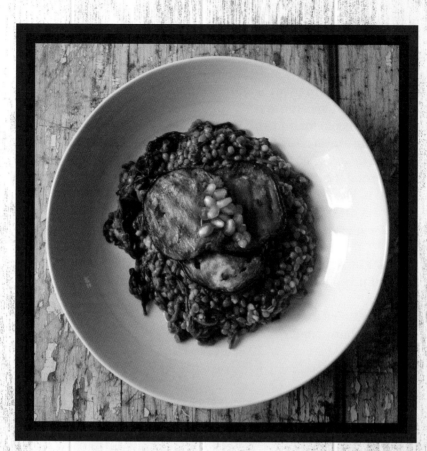

CHAPTER 1:
The Secret Trimester
(weeks 1–12)

Eating Well in the Secret Trimester

During the first trimester a life is being created. During the second and third trimesters a life is being grown. This goes some way towards explaining the feelings of exhaustion some women experience during the first trimester. It's also why mum-to-be may find herself craving carbs carbs carbs, to give herself the energy boost she needs. Food-wise, the first trimester can be a tricky time. True, it's not always quite like the films where mum-to-be suddenly runs out of a meeting due to morning sickness, but it may be surprising to suddenly have no appetite for the healthy greens she was eating just a few weeks before. My wife, for example, couldn't bear the sight of an avocado (her favourite food) during the first 12 weeks of pregnancy.

Even if morning sickness isn't an issue (and it is in around 75 per cent of pregnancies), what with mum-to-be experiencing massive hormonal changes early on in the first trimester, it's totally normal for appetites to change. Add to that the strains of modern life and the fact that a lot of people keep pregnancies a secret in the first trimester, eating well just isn't top of the list — getting to the end of each day is.

As is true of any time really, it's important that mum-to-be listens to what her body is telling her, not what anyone else is. She may well be craving just carbs and may only want bland food. There is absolutely nothing wrong with this and if that's how she feels, go with it. Some people want nothing more than mac 'n' cheese (see page 24), poached eggs (see page 20) and meatballs and mash (see page 34) on repeat. In fact, you could call this time the beige-food trimester too!

As long as mum-to-be is taking her recommended vitamin supplements, it's totally normal to just respond to what her body is telling her and eat the foods she wants. However, there are certain types of food that are really good to eat in the secret trimester and this is what this chapter focuses on. If mum-to-be is feeling great and has an appetite for a wide variety of foods, then brilliant, go wild. If, however, she isn't, this chapter will give some ideas on how to incorporate those foods.

It's also worth saying that every pregnancy is different for every woman. In her first pregnancy my wife couldn't even sniff a vegetable for the first trimester; second pregnancy first trimester, all she wanted to eat was a tomato and onion salad every day. Go figure!

What to focus on

>> **COMPLEX CARBS:** If carb-heavy, bland foods are what mum-to-be wants to eat then she should eat them. However, with a few simple changes she can really increase her nutrient intake. Instead of white bread, try switching it for some wholegrain bread with lots of seeds. Instead of white potatoes, she could eat more sweet potatoes (or cauliflower mash) and swap white rice and pasta for brown rice and whole-wheat pasta. All these foods contain lots of vitamins and minerals such as calcium, iron, B vitamins and potassium, which are really good for mum-to-be, and for baby's development. They are also great sources of fibre, which helps her to not feel bloated or heavy.

>> **PROTEIN:** As well as wanting carb-heavy foods, it's quite normal to crave protein for the extra energy kick. Protein is also essential for mum-to-be and baby's growth and development, so portions of lean meats (chicken, turkey, pork and beef), fish, eggs, yogurt, cheese, tofu, nuts, beans and pulses/legumes are super.

>> **FOLATE:** Folic acid (or folate as it's called when it naturally occurs in food) is an essential nutrient in pregnancy, as it prevents neural tube defects in baby. Mum-to-be's supplements will contain all the folate she needs but it is also found in high quantities in green leafy vegetables (spinach, kale, cabbage), broccoli, peas, avocado, peppers, chickpeas/garbanzo beans, lentils, eggs, nuts and seeds, bananas and citrus fruits.

You'll find that all of the recipes in the secret trimester focus on helping mum-to-be incorporate more wholegrains, protein, folate and other essential nutrients into her diet. In some pregnancies spicier foods are craved early on, so there are a few recipes that include spices and chillies. If that's not the case, however, just remove them.

SPOTLIGHT:

Six Awesome Folate-Rich Pesto Recipes

* EACH RECIPE MAKES APPROX. 12 ICE CUBES OF PESTO *
* BATCH-COOK ME! *
* FAMILY-FRIENDLY, JUST LEAVE OUT THE SALT *
* VEGETARIAN/VEGAN IF YOU LEAVE OUT THE PARMESAN *

It's very common in the first trimester for vegetables to be something mum-to-be can't stomach or has literally no appetite for. While leaving out vegetables in this early period isn't a big deal (as long as you're taking supplements) we can make them a bit more appealing. Making your own pesto is a great way of getting in a relatively large quantity of veg (folate-rich greens too, so great for the first trimester). Pesto is so versatile. Plus, it's totally freezable, so make a big batch, freeze in ice-cube trays and then you have a ready-made supply to use as and when you want.

>> **SERVING SUGGESTIONS:** Pesto isn't just for stirring into pasta. Here are a few ways you can use pesto to not only add flavour to dishes but improve their nutritional content too: stir a teaspoon or two into any soup; spread it over some chicken, lamb, fish or vegetables before grilling or roasting; stuff inside a chicken breast; stir into a bowl of boiled Jersey potatoes; use as a salad dressing; or simply spread it thickly on some wholegrain toast.

>> **STORAGE:** Store pesto in the refrigerator in an air-tight container with a thin layer of olive oil on top. The oil acts like a seal and stops the pesto from going bad. It will keep for around five days. My preference, however, is to make a big batch and freeze it in ice-cube trays, then remove from the tray and store loose in freezer bags. It will last around three months this way. Just leave it out to defrost for about an hour before using, then add directly to your chosen dish.

>> **MIX IT UP:** While I've used cheese in a few of the recipes in this chapter, feel free to leave it out or replace it with a vegan cheese substitute. Experiment with alternative ingredients such as kale, courgette/zucchini, cauliflower and so on too. Leave out any nuts mentioned too, if you have an allergy.

All recipes make 12 ice cubes. Two cubes serve one person. Some recipes require 20 minutes' roasting but otherwise all prep time is minimal.

The Classic: Basil, Pine Nut & Parmesan Pesto

Ingredients

60g/2¼oz/½ cup pine nuts ✳ 100g/3½oz fresh basil (including stalks) ✳ 2 garlic cloves ✳ 60g/2¼oz/½ cup grated Parmesan cheese ✳ 100ml/3½fl oz/scant ½ cup olive oil ✳ Salt and pepper, to taste

METHOD

1 Lightly toast the pine nuts in a hot, dry frying pan for a few minutes until they start to smell nutty.

2 Blend together the basil, garlic, Parmesan, pine nuts and approximately two-thirds of the oil in a food processor.

3 Taste, then season and add more oil, if needed, to achieve your preferred texture.

Roasted Red Pepper, Tomato & Almond Pesto

Ingredients

2 red peppers, core removed, deseeded and sliced ✳ 2 large tomatoes, sliced ✳ 3 garlic cloves, unpeeled ✳ 2 tablespoons olive oil ✳ 60g/2¼oz/½ cup almonds ✳ Salt and pepper, to taste

METHOD

1 Preheat the oven to 180°C/350°F/ Gas 4.

2 Put the peppers, tomatoes and garlic into a roasting pan, season and drizzle one teaspoon of olive oil over. Roast for 20 minutes. Add the almonds to the pan halfway through the cooking time.

3 Remove the pan from the oven. Squeeze the roasted garlic from their skins, which you can discard, then blend everything together in a food processor, along with the remaining olive oil. As the tomatoes have so much liquid, you don't need as much olive oil as in the other recipes.

Rocket, Walnut & Parmesan Pesto

Ingredients

60g/2¼oz/⅓ cup walnuts ✳ 100g/3½oz rocket/arugula ✳ 60g/2¼oz/½ cup Parmesan cheese ✳ 2 garlic cloves ✳ 100ml/3½fl oz/ scant ½ cup olive oil ✳ Salt and pepper, to taste

METHOD

1 Lightly toast the walnuts in a hot, dry frying pan for a few minutes until they start to smell nutty.

2 Blend the rocket/arugula, Parmesan, garlic, walnuts and approximately two-thirds of the olive oil in a food processor, then season and add more olive oil to taste.

Pea, Pistachio & Mint Pesto

Ingredients

100g/3½oz/½ cup frozen peas ✳ 25g/1oz mint leaves ✳ 60g/2¼oz/⅓ cup shelled pistachios ✳ 3 tablespoons olive oil ✳ Salt and pepper, to taste

METHOD

1 Place the peas in a bowl, pour boiling water over them and leave to stand for a few minutes.

2 Lightly toast the pistachios in a hot, dry frying pan for a few minutes until they start to smell nutty.

3 Drain the peas then blend everything together in a food processor and season to taste.

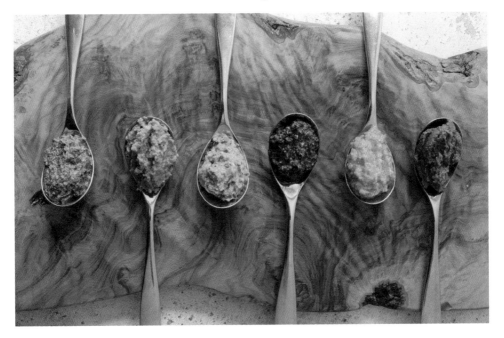

Broccoli, Spinach & Cashew Nut Pesto

Ingredients

1 head of broccoli, cut into florets ✳ 60g/2¼oz/ ⅓ cup cashew nuts ✳ 30g/1oz spinach ✳ 100ml/3½fl oz/scant ½ cup olive oil ✳ Salt and pepper, to taste

METHOD

1 Place the broccoli florets into a pan of boiling water for 2–3 minutes, then drain.

2 Lightly toast the cashew nuts in a hot, dry frying pan for a few minutes until they start to smell nutty.

3 Blend two-thirds of the olive oil, the cashew nuts, spinach and broccoli together in a food processor, adding more olive oil and salt and pepper to taste.

Beetroot & Walnut Pesto

Ingredients

250g/9oz pre-cooked beetroot/beets, thinly sliced ✳ 60g/2¼oz/⅓ cup walnuts ✳ Juice of 1 lemon ✳ 4 tablespoons olive oil ✳ Salt and pepper, to taste

METHOD

1 Preheat the oven to 180°C/350°F/ Gas 4.

2 Place the sliced beetroot/beets in a roasting pan and roast for 20 minutes. Halfway through the cooking time, add the walnuts. Remove the pan from the oven and tip everything into a food processor.

3 Blend with the lemon juice and olive oil, then season to taste.

Making your own pesto is a great way of getting a relatively large amount of folate-rich greens into a dish

Spanish Tortilla with Sweet Potato & Peas

Using sweet potatoes instead of traditional white potatoes, as well as adding peas, immediately ramps up the nutritional value of this dish. It's great for brunch or a light lunch — or if mum-to-be isn't feeling like eating that much. Cut it into squares, keep in the fridge and snack on it over the next day or so.

SERVES 2, plus leftovers for lunch the next day
Prep time: 10 minutes
Cook time: 30 minutes

* VEGETARIAN
* FAMILY-FRIENDLY, just leave out the salt

Ingredients

A knob of butter (or a plant-based alternative)
2 sweet potatoes, peeled and diced into 1cm cubes
100g/3½oz/½ cup frozen peas
8–10 eggs
Salt

>> **MIX IT UP:**
* Loads of possibilities here: add in some diced onion, kale, spinach, bacon, chorizo, mozzarella, olives, sun-dried tomatoes, and so on.
* Top with grated cheese or eat it in a crusty baguette. I like to cover my tortilla with hot sauce and eat it alongside a green salad.

1 Melt the butter in a frying pan (minimum 24cm/9½ in) over a medium heat. Add the sweet potatoes along with a pinch of salt and cook for 6–8 minutes until they begin to soften. Add the frozen peas, stir and remove from the heat.

2 Crack the eggs into a large bowl and mix well. Add the sweet potato and pea mixture to the bowl, stir well, then tip everything back into the pan (adding a little butter to the pan first if you need). Cook over a medium heat for around 15 minutes until the top of the tortilla begins to solidify. Run a spatula occasionally around the sides of the tortilla to ensure it doesn't stick.

3 Remove the pan from the heat and cover with a chopping board. Flip the pan over so the tortilla is on the board, then slide it back into the pan. Cook for a further 3–4 minutes.

4 Remove the tortilla from the pan and either eat straight away or leave to cool, then refrigerate. Eat within 24–48 hours.

Poached Egg, Chorizo, Red Pepper & Sweet Potato Hash

A hearty brunch made all the better by mixing the gooey egg yolk in with the delicious sweet potato and chorizo. This dish packs some heat and is full of folate, protein, healthy carbs and vitamins — ideal for a first trimester bowl of comfort food.

SERVES 2–3
Prep time: 10 minutes
Cook time: 15 minutes

Ingredients

2–3 sweet potatoes, peeled and diced
1 teaspoon olive oil
1 onion, diced
150g/5½oz chorizo, sliced
1 red pepper, cored, deseeded
    and diced
4–6 eggs
1 teaspoon white wine vinegar
    (to cook the poached eggs)
2–3 spring onions/scallions,
    thinly sliced
1 green chilli, diced
A few leaves of parsley, chopped
Salt

> **>> MIX IT UP:**
> * Swap the sweet potatoes for squash or pumpkin.
> * Replace the poached eggs with fried.
> * Leave out the chorizo but replace with a teaspoon of smoked paprika to keep the heat.

1 Tip the sweet potatoes into a pan of lightly salted boiling water and cook for 4–5 minutes. Drain and leave to steam-dry.

2 Heat the oil in a frying pan over a medium heat. Add the onion and a pinch of salt and cook for 2–3 minutes. Add the chorizo and red pepper and cook for a further 2–3 minutes.

3 Add the sweet potatoes to the pan and mix well. Gently crush the potatoes with the back of a wooden spoon just to squish everything down a bit and create a hash.

4 To make the poached eggs, bring a deep, wide pan of water to the boil. Reduce to a simmer, add the vinegar and stir gently to create a circular effect, this helps wrap the egg white around the yolk. Crack the eggs from a low height one or two at a time into the pan and cook for 3–4 minutes. Remove with a slotted spoon and place on some paper towels to remove the excess water.

5 Spoon the hash into bowls. Top with the poached eggs, spring onions/scallions, diced chilli and parsley before serving.

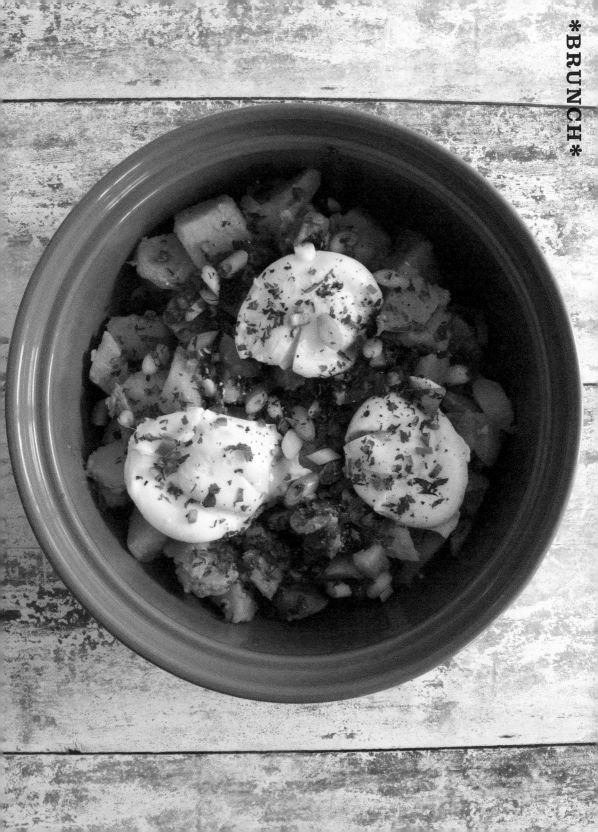

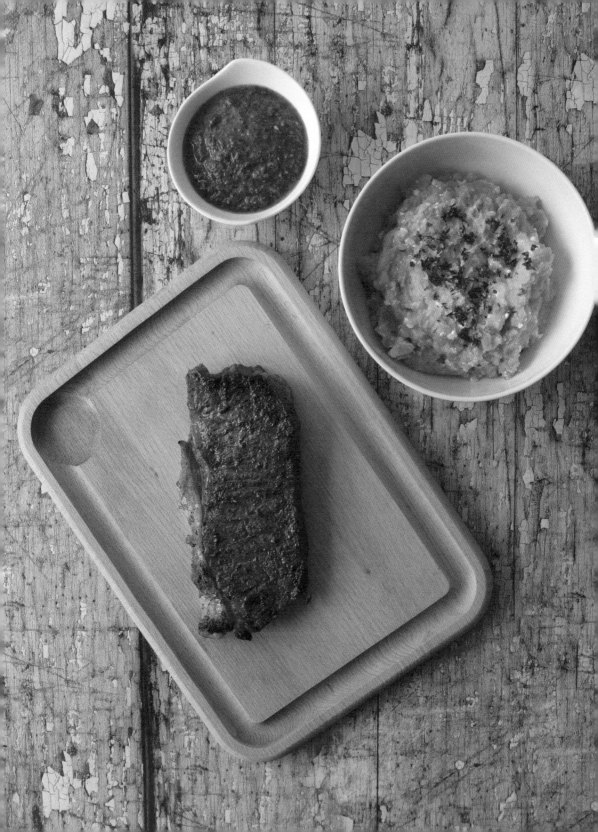

Sirloin Steak with Sweet Potato Feta Mash & Chimichurri

A steak is an excellent choice in the first trimester because of its high iron content. Feta is a great source of calcium, swapping standard mash for sweet potato mash increases mum-to-be's nutrient intake and the homemade chimichurri provides a good dose of folate and other vitamins.

SERVES 2
Prep time: 10 minutes
Cook time: 10 minutes

Ingredients

3–4 sweet potatoes, peeled and sliced
100g/3½oz/⅔ cup feta cheese (optional)
a bunch of coriander/cilantro, roughly chopped
a bunch of parsley, roughly chopped
1 shallot, roughly chopped
1 garlic clove
1 green chilli, deseeded
5 tablespoons olive oil, plus extra for frying
1 teaspoon red wine vinegar
2 sirloin steaks, about 200g/7oz each
Salt and pepper

1 Tip the sweet potatoes into a pan of lightly salted water, bring to the boil and cook for 5 minutes. Drain and then mash with the feta. Keep warm.

2 To make the chimichurri, place the coriander/cilantro and parsley (stalks included) in a food processor. Blend along with the shallot, garlic, chilli, olive oil, red wine vinegar and a pinch of salt.

3 Heat a little oil in a frying pan over a medium heat. Season the steaks and cook to your preference (2 minutes each side for medium-rare, 3 for medium and 4 for well done). Allow the meat to rest for 5 minutes and then serve alongside the mashed sweet potato and chimichurri.

>> **MIX IT UP:**
* If you don't fancy beef, chimichurri works well with either pork or cauliflower steaks.
* Swap the feta for grated Cheddar, Gouda or vegan cheese.

Hearty Mac 'N' Cheese with Butternut Squash & Sage Crisps

This is not just delicious, warming and satisfying for when mum-to-be craves carbs carbs carbs, but it also contains some fantastically healthy squash and sage. The whole-wheat pasta contains fibre and other lovely nutrients. My wife ate this a lot in her first trimester. Make a big batch to keep in the freezer or transform the leftovers into mac 'n' cheese "arancini" (see page 178). Bookmark this for later on in pregnancy when you're batchcooking too.

SERVES 2, plus a few portions for the freezer

Prep time: 15 minutes

Cook time: 35 minutes

✱ BATCH-COOK ME!

✱ FAMILY-FRIENDLY, just leave out the salt and sage crisps for under-1s

✱ VEGETARIAN

Ingredients

1 butternut squash, peeled and cut into small cubes

2 teaspoons olive oil

500g/1lb 2oz/5 cups whole-wheat macaroni

50g/1¾oz unsalted butter

50g/1¾oz/⅓ cup plain/all-purpose white flour

600ml/21fl oz/2½ cups full-fat/whole milk

200g/7oz/1½ cups grated Cheddar cheese

100g/3¾oz/¾ cup Parmesan cheese, grated

2 garlic cloves, crushed

8–10 sage leaves

Salt and pepper

1 Preheat the oven to 180°C/350°F/Gas 4.

2 Place the squash in a roasting pan, drizzle with about a teaspoon of olive oil, season and roast for 15 minutes until softened. Meanwhile, cook the macaroni in salted boiling water for 2 minutes less than the packet instructions state, then drain.

3 Melt the butter in a saucepan over a medium heat and then add the flour. Allow to cook for 30 seconds before whisking well. Add the milk in slowly, whisking continuously until you have a thick sauce. Cook for a further minute without stirring. Add the Cheddar and half of the Parmesan and mix well. Finally, add the garlic into the mix.

4 Tip the macaroni into an ovenproof dish along with the squash. Pour over the cheese sauce and stir well. Bake for 20 minutes.

5 Meanwhile, heat a little olive oil in a pan and fry the sage leaves for about a minute on each side until they become crispy. Remove and place on some paper towels to drain.

6 Remove the macaroni cheese from the oven when the top is bubbling and golden. Serve in bowls, topped with the sage crisps.

>> **MIX IT UP:**
* Blend half of the squash and add to the cheese sauce.
* Swap the squash for pumpkin (especially at Halloween), courgette/zucchini, parsnip or carrot.
* Some diced bacon also works well.

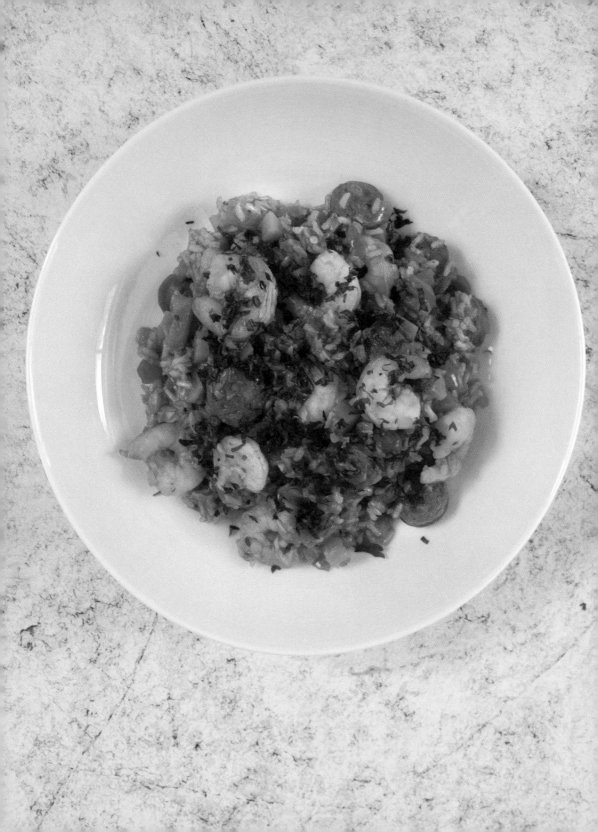

Prawn & Chorizo Jambalaya

Another dish that's packed full of bold flavours and is great to tuck into at the end of a long day. Red peppers are packed full of vitamins, including folate, and prawns/shrimp are little parcels of protein — so all in all, a great first trimester dish! This one is perfect for batch-cooking and freezing.

SERVES 4, plus some
    for the freezer
Prep time: 15 minutes
Cook time: 35 minutes

✱ BATCH-COOK ME!
✱ FAMILY-FRIENDLY

Ingredients

1 teaspoon olive oil
1 onion, diced
1 teaspoon cayenne pepper
1 teaspoon dried oregano
1 teaspoon smoked paprika
1 teaspoon dried thyme
2 garlic cloves, finely chopped
250g/9oz chorizo, sliced
2 red peppers, cored, deseeded
    and diced
2 carrots, diced
400g/14oz/2 cups brown rice
1 x 400g/14oz can of chopped
    tomatoes
600ml/21fl oz/scant 2½ cups
    vegetable stock
300g/10½oz raw peeled king
    prawns/shrimp
A few parsley sprigs, chopped

1 Heat the oil in a wide frying pan over a medium heat. Add the onion and fry for 2–3 minutes. Add the cayenne pepper, oregano, paprika and thyme, stir and cook for another 2 minutes.

2 Add the garlic to the pan, along with the chorizo. Cook for 3–4 minutes.

3 Add the peppers and carrots and cook for 3 more minutes. Add the rice, chopped tomatoes and stock. Bring to the boil, then reduce to a simmer and cook for 20 minutes. The pan must be covered or the rice won't cook so quickly.

4 Finally, add the prawns/shrimp and cook for about 3 minutes until they turn pink. Sprinkle over the parsley and serve.

>> **MIX IT UP:**
✱ For a chorizo or prawn/shrimp jambalaya, simply leave out one and double the quantity of the other.
✱ For a vegan option, swap out the chorizo and prawns for butter/ lima beans.

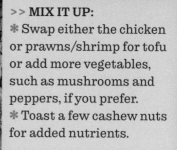

>> **MIX IT UP:**
* Swap either the chicken
or prawns/shrimp for tofu
or add more vegetables,
such as mushrooms and
peppers, if you prefer.
* Toast a few cashew nuts
for added nutrients.

Nasi Goreng

This is perfect first trimester food. The heat and salt hit those early pregnancy cravings, the rice ticks the carbs box, and the chicken, prawns and eggs are full of protein. It's also great for hiding veg.

SERVES 2

Prep time: 15 minutes

Cook time: 20 minutes

Ingredients

250g/9oz/1¼ cups brown basmati rice

4 tablespoons olive oil

4 eggs

1 onion, half thinly sliced and half diced

200g/7oz raw peeled prawns/shrimp

1 chicken breast, diced into 1cm/½in pieces

3 garlic cloves, finely chopped

1 carrot, diced

100g/3½oz green beans, chopped

1 red chilli, deseeded and diced

4 tablespoons soy sauce

1 tablespoon honey

1 tablespoon sriracha or other hot sauce

1 large tomato, thinly sliced

2.5cm/1in piece of cucumber, thinly sliced

2 spring onions/scallions, thinly sliced

1 Cook the rice as per the packet instructions. Drain, then allow to cool. Set aside.

2 Meanwhile, heat a tablespoon of the oil in a frying pan over medium heat. Whisk 2 of the eggs in a bowl, then pour into the pan. Move the pan around to spread the eggs out evenly to create a thin omelette. It will only take a few minutes to cook. Remove from the pan and set aside.

3 Heat a tablespoon of the oil in the pan and add the sliced onions. Cook for 7−8 minutes until golden and crispy. Remove and set aside.

4 Add the prawns to the pan and cook for 2−3 minutes until pink. Remove and set aside.

5 Heat another tablespoon of oil in the pan, add the diced onions and cook for 2−3 minutes. Add the chicken and cook for 5 minutes. Add the garlic, carrot, green beans and chilli.

6 Mix the soy sauce, honey and sriracha together in a small bowl, then add to the pan along with the rice. Slice the omelette into small pieces and add to the pan along with the cooked prawns. Cook for 2 minutes.

7 Fry the remaining 2 eggs in a separate pan in the remaining tablespoon of oil over medium heat.

8 Divide the nasi goreng between 2 plates. Scatter over the tomato and cucumber. Top each with a fried egg and garnish with the crispy onions and spring onions/scallions.

Minestrone

A big bowl of chunky soup is sometimes just what the doctor ordered. Minestrone is full of so many fantastic vegetables, pulses and greens and is also a delicious carb-heavy, warming broth that's ready in no time at all. Perfect for a first trimester evening.

SERVES 2, plus lots for
the freezer
Prep time: 10 minutes
Cook time: 25 minutes

✳ BATCH-COOK ME!
✳ VEGETARIAN/VEGAN
✳ FAMILY-FRIENDLY,
just leave out the salt

Ingredients

1 tablespoon olive oil
1 onion, diced
2 garlic cloves, crushed
1 teaspoon dried thyme
1 teaspoon dried sage
2 large carrots, diced
2 celery stalks, diced
1 x 400g/14oz can of chopped
tomatoes
1 tablespoon tomato purée/paste
600ml/21fl oz/2½ cups vegetable
stock (use baby-friendly stock if
cooking for babies)
200g/7oz small pasta, such as
farfalline, ditalini, orzo or macaroni
1 x 400g/14oz can of butter/lima
beans, drained
Large handful of kale, tough stalks
removed, roughly chopped

1 Heat a tablespoon of oil in a large frying pan over a medium heat. Add the onion and fry for 2–3 minutes. Add the garlic along with the thyme and sage. Add the carrots and celery and cook for 5 minutes.

2 Add the chopped tomatoes, tomato purée/paste and stock to the pan, bring to a simmer, cover and cook for 15 minutes.

3 Cook the pasta as per the packet instructions. Drain then set aside.

4 Add the butter/lima beans to the pan along with the kale. Add the pasta and cook for a further 2 minutes before serving.

> > **MIX IT UP:**
✳ Add some Parmesan or other grated cheese at the end.
✳ Swap the butter/lima beans for cannellini or borlotti.
✳ Add some brown rice instead of pasta, if you prefer, or serve with some crusty bread.

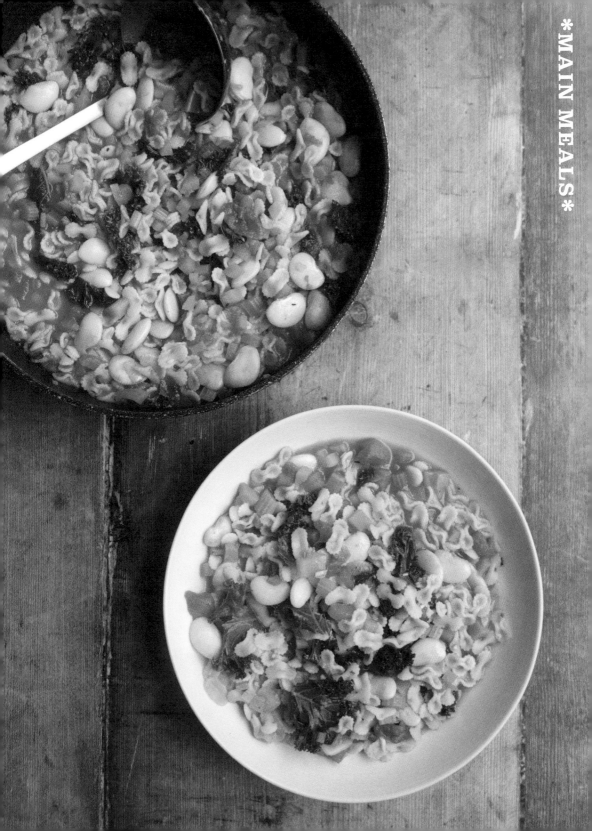

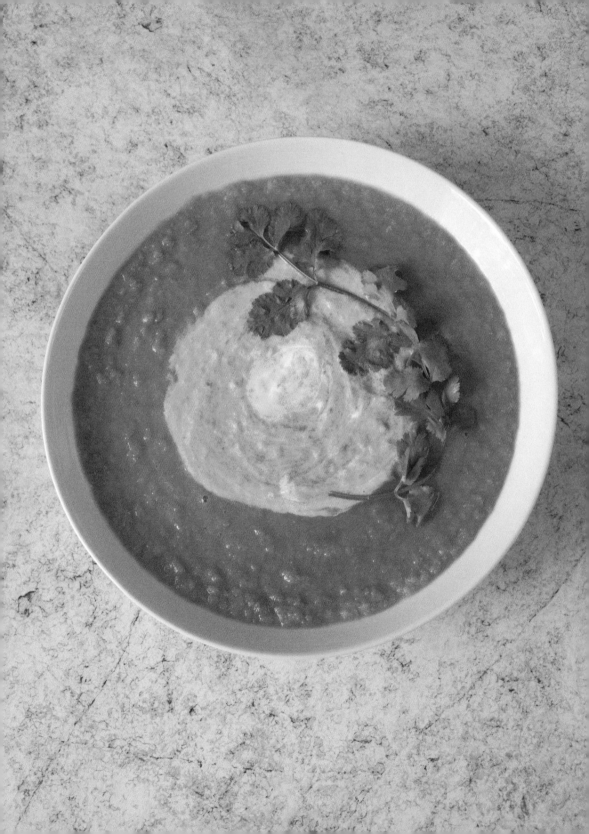

Carrot, Lentil, Cumin & Coriander Soup

An easy way to increase vegetable intake is with a simple warming soup, especially if this time occurs over winter. (For some chilled soup recipes to have when it's warmer, see page 58.) Not only are soups straightforward to make and a wonderful way to use up pretty much any vegetable in the refrigerator, they're also great for batch-cooking and freezing. If mum-to-be wants to increase her nutrient intake but the thought of crunching vegetables makes her stomach turn, blending them into soups is a great solution.

SERVES 2
Prep time: 5 minutes
Cook time: 20 minutes

* BATCH-COOK ME!
* FAMILY-FRIENDLY,
    just leave out the salt
* VEGETARIAN/VEGAN

Ingredients

1 teaspoon olive oil
1 onion, diced
1 teaspoon ground cumin
1 teaspoon ground coriander
600ml/20fl oz/2½ cups vegetable
    stock (use baby-friendly stock if
    cooking for babies)
8 carrots, chopped
1 x 400g/14oz can of green lentils,
    drained
A few coriander/cilantro sprigs,
    leaves chopped

1 Heat the oil in a frying pan over a low heat. Add the onion and cook for 2–3 minutes. Add the cumin and ground coriander, mix well, and cook for a few more minutes. Turn off the heat and set aside.

2 In a saucepan, bring the vegetable stock to the boil. Add the carrots along with the cooked onion and spices, bring back to the boil and simmer for 10 minutes.

3 Add the lentils, cook for another 2 minutes, then blend to your chosen consistency, either in a blender or using a hand-held/immersion blender. Sprinkle over the fresh coriander/ cilantro before serving.

>> **MIX IT UP:**
* Stir in some cooked whole-wheat pasta or brown rice for a more filling meal.
* Add a dollop of yogurt (pictured), a splash of coconut milk, a spoonful of pesto, chunks of cooked sausage or chorizo, croutons or – my favourite – add a few cubes of cheese to the soup and let them melt.
* Try Parmesan crisps! Grate Parmesan, arrange in small discs on baking paper and bake for 10 minutes at 180°C/350°F/Gas 4.

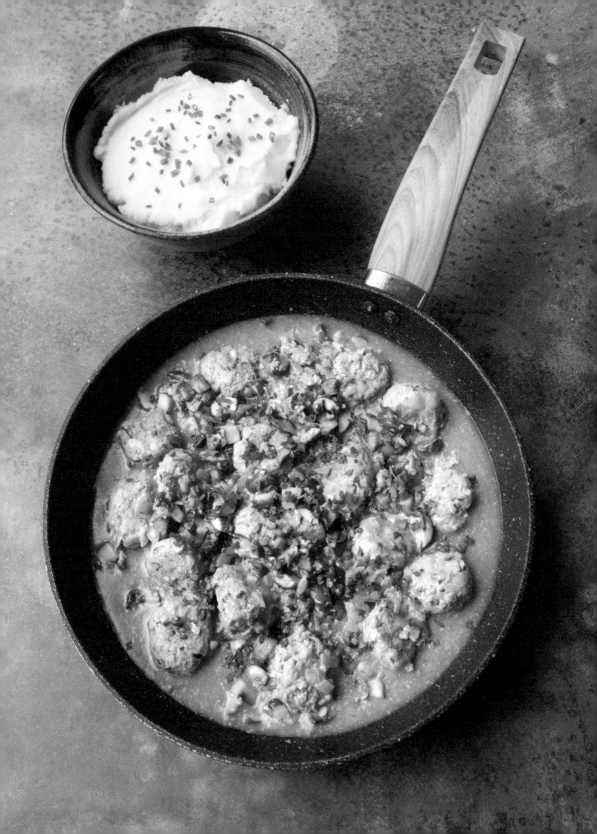

Pork, Courgette & Cheese Meatballs with Cauliflower Purée & Mushroom Gravy

This is one of my most popular dishes and a real bowl of comfort. Making your own meatballs lets you hide some vegetables in them, but shop-bought are fine too. Swapping mash for cauliflower is a game-changer. One portion of cauliflower contains three-quarters of the vitamin C you need in one day and I also think it tastes better!

SERVES 2

Prep time: 10 minutes, plus 30 minutes chilling time

Cook time: 20 minutes

✱ FAMILY-FRIENDLY, just leave out the salt

Ingredients

2 shallots, diced

1 courgette/zucchini, grated

50g/1¾oz/⅓ cup Cheddar cheese, grated

1 egg, beaten

400g/14oz minced/ground pork

2 tablespoons olive oil

1 head of cauliflower, cut into florets

a knob of butter (or a plant-based alternative)

2 tablespoons full-fat/whole milk (or a plant-based alternative)

1 garlic clove, finely chopped

200g/7oz/3 cups chestnut/cremini mushrooms, thinly sliced

1 tablespoon plain/all-purpose white flour (or any alternative)

200ml/7fl oz/scant 1 cup beef stock

A few parsley sprigs, leaves chopped

Salt

1 Place half of the shallots, the grated courgette/zucchini, Cheddar, egg and pork in a bowl. Season with salt, then mix well with your hands. Roll the mixture into golf-ball-sized balls; you should have enough for about 16. Place on a plate, cover with cling film/plastic wrap then refrigerate for 30 minutes.

2 Heat a tablespoon of oil in a frying pan over a medium heat. Add the meatballs and cook, turning regularly, for about 10 minutes. Allow the meatballs space to cook; you may need to cook in two batches. When cooked, set aside.

3 Cook the cauliflower in a pan of boiling water for 3–4 minutes. Drain then place in a food processor or blender along with the butter and milk. Blend to a purée consistency.

4 Heat the remaining tablespoon of oil in the frying pan. Add the remaining shallots and cook for a few minutes. Then add in the garlic, stir in the mushrooms and cook for a few more minutes. Mix the flour into the beef stock and pour into the pan. Add the meatballs back in and cook for 2–3 minutes.

5 Spoon the purée onto two plates. Add the meatballs on top, spoon over the mushrooms and gravy, and finally sprinkle with parsley.

Ramen Three Ways: Salmon, Tofu & Beef

Ramen is an excellent dish that's so easy to make at home. Sweetcorn and pak choi/bok choy are often-overlooked sources of folate. The combination of these with whole-wheat noodles and protein like beef, salmon or tofu makes a great first trimester meal.

SERVES 2
Prep time: 15 minutes
Cook time: 20 minutes

✳ FAMILY-FRIENDLY,
just leave out the salt

Ingredients

1 x 200g/7oz pack of tofu, cut into
    bite-size cubes, or 1 salmon fillet
    (about 200g/7oz), or 1 sirloin
    steak (about 200g/7oz)
2 teaspoons soy sauce, plus 1 extra
    teaspoon if using salmon
2 eggs
200g/7oz whole-wheat noodles
500ml/17fl oz/2 cups vegetable
    stock
3 tablespoons miso paste
5cm/2in piece of fresh root ginger,
    peeled and finely grated
1 garlic clove, finely chopped
100g/3½oz/½ cup frozen sweetcorn
200g/7oz pak choi/bok choy, sliced
3–4 spring onions/scallions, sliced
2–3 teaspoons sesame seeds
Salt and pepper

1 Heat the oven to 180°C/350°F/Gas 4 if you're using tofu or salmon. For the tofu, place the cubes on a baking sheet and cook for 15 minutes. For the salmon, place on a baking sheet, sprinkle over a teaspoon of the soy sauce and cook for 8 minutes.

2 If using steak, season and cook to your liking (2 minutes each side for medium-rare, 3 for medium, 4 for well done). Let rest for 5 minutes.

3 Cook the eggs in a pan of boiling water for around 5–6 minutes. Drain then leave in a bowl of iced water (to stop them cooking).

4 Cook the noodles as per the packet instructions, then drain and set aside.

5 Pour the stock into a saucepan and bring to the boil over a medium heat. Stir in the miso and 1 teaspoon of the soy sauce. Add the ginger, garlic, sweetcorn and pak choi/bok choy and cook for a further minute.

6 Peel the eggs, cut them in half, put them in a bowl and pour over the remaining soy sauce.

7 Assemble: divide the noodles into 2 bowls. Add the tofu, salmon or beef. Place the eggs on top. Remove the pak choi from the broth and add to the bowls. Spoon in the broth. Finally, sprinkle with spring onions/scallions and sesame seeds before serving.

>> **MIX IT UP:**
* Add either a little
fresh chilli or a spoonful
of sriracha for some
extra heat.
* Marinate the beef,
salmon or tofu in a little
honey and soy sauce
before cooking.
* Add in mushrooms,
peas or carrots for more
vegetables.

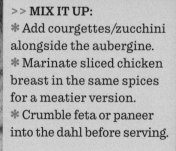

>> **MIX IT UP:**

✱ Add courgettes/zucchini alongside the aubergine.

✱ Marinate sliced chicken breast in the same spices for a meatier version.

✱ Crumble feta or paneer into the dahl before serving.

Spiced Aubergine, Spinach & Green Lentil Dhal

A hearty dhal tends to go down very well in early pregnancy as it's so easy to eat. When you cook the lentils in the spices and stock, they take on such a delicious flavour and they go so well with the texture of the vitamin- and folate-rich aubergine/eggplant. Top with some pomegranate seeds for a burst of sweetness and vitamin C.

SERVES 2
Prep time: 10 minutes
Cook time: 30 minutes

* BATCH-COOK ME!
* VEGETARIAN/VEGAN
* FAMILY-FRIENDLY,
   just leave out the salt

Ingredients

1 large aubergine/eggplant
3 tablespoons olive oil
1 tablespoon garam masala
1 tablespoon ground cinnamon
1 tablespoon ground coriander
1 tablespoon ground cumin
1 onion, diced
3 garlic cloves, finely chopped
2.5cm/1in piece of fresh root ginger,
   peeled and grated
2 x 400g/14oz can of green lentils,
   drained
500ml/17fl oz/2 cups vegetable
   stock
2 large handfuls of baby spinach
a handful of coriander/cilantro leaves
2 tablespoons pomegranate seeds

1 Cut the top and bottom off the aubergine/eggplant, then slice into 1cm/½in discs. Drizzle with 2 tablespoons of the oil and sprinkle with a pinch of each of the spices. Cook on a griddle/grill pan over a medium heat for 12–15 minutes, turning once. You may need to do this in batches.

2 While the aubergine is cooking, heat a tablespoon of the oil in a frying pan over a medium heat. Add the onion and the remaining spices and mix well. Cook for around 3 minutes. Add the garlic and ginger to the pan and cook for a further minute.

3 Add the green lentils and vegetable stock. Bring to the boil, turn the heat down and simmer for 15 minutes.

4 Towards the end of the cooking time, add the spinach and stir until wilted. Divide the dhal between 2 bowls, then top with the aubergine, a few coriander/cilantro leaves and pomegranate seeds before serving.

Sweet Potato & Pea Tartiflette

Tartiflette is a gorgeous French dish of potatoes, cream, cheese and lardons. My wife inhaled a tartiflette in a restaurant in her first trimester, so I created a slightly healthier version. I've upped the nutrients with sweet potatoes and peas, swapped Reblochon for Gruyère and made it lighter by using milk rather than cream.

SERVES 2
Prep time: 10 minutes
Cook time: 40 minutes

Ingredients

2 large Maris Piper/russet potatoes
   (or similar), peeled and diced into
   2cm /¾in cubes
a knob of butter (or a plant-based
   alternative)
1 onion, diced
1 garlic clove, crushed
2 large sweet potatoes, peeled and
   diced into 2cm/¾in cubes
6–8 thick-cut bacon rashers/slices,
   diced
100g/3½oz/½ cup frozen peas
400ml/14fl oz/1⅔ cups full-fat/
   whole milk (or a plant-based
   alternative)
100g/3½oz/¾ cup Cheddar cheese,
   grated
200g/7oz/1½ cups Gruyère cheese,
   sliced
Salt

1 Preheat the oven to 180°C/350°F/Gas 4.

2 Cook the white potatoes in a pan of lightly salted water for 7–8 minutes until soft. Drain and leave to cool.

3 Melt the butter in a pan over a medium heat. Add the onion along with a pinch of salt, and cook for 5 minutes.

4 Add the garlic and sweet potatoes and cook for another 5 minutes. Mix in the bacon and cook for a further 2 minutes. Add the frozen peas and the white potatoes and mix everything together well. Spoon the mixture into a baking dish.

5 Pour the milk into the empty pan and gently warm it over a low heat for a few minutes. Stir in the Cheddar.

6 Pour the milk over the potato mix. Scatter over the Gruyère, then bake for 20 mins or so until the cheese is golden and melting.

> > **MIX IT UP:**
> ✳ Try adding some nutmeg or a spoonful of mustard to the milk for a hint of spice.
> ✳ Swap the bacon for chorizo, but cook the chorizo separately before adding.
> ✳ For a non-meat version, broccoli or cauliflower work well instead of the bacon.
> ✳ Plant-based milks and vegan cheese can also be used.

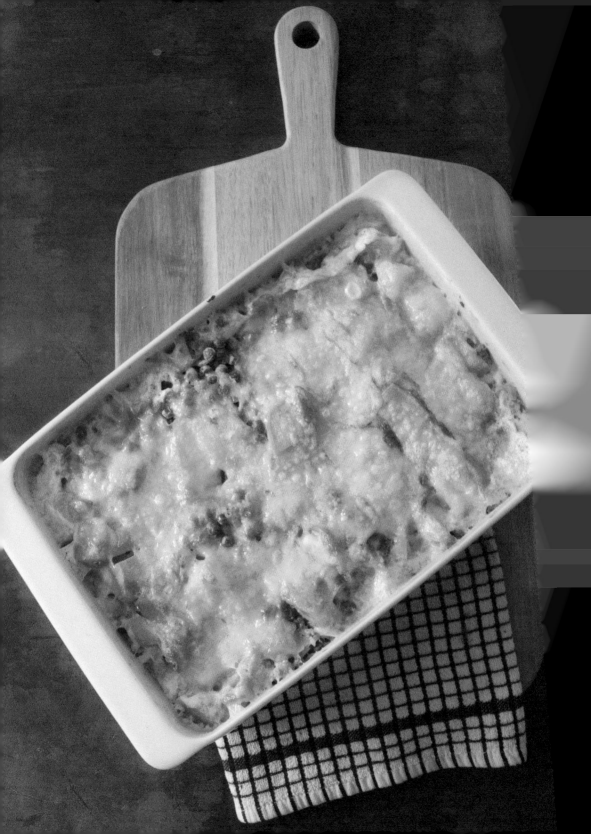

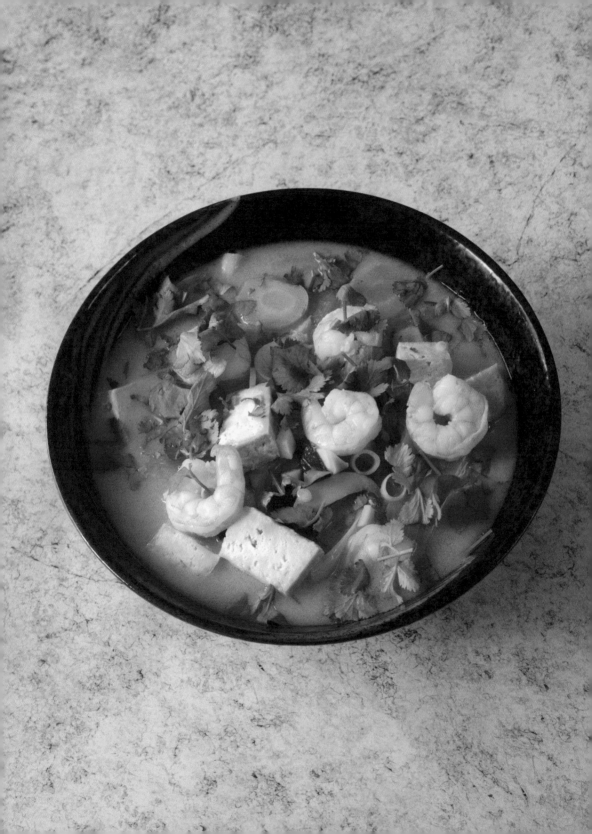

Thai Coconut & Lemongrass Soup with King Prawns & Tofu

Coconut milk is so delicious when mixed with ginger, chilli, lemongrass and lime in this Thai soup. Add your choice of protein and some folate-rich pak choi/bok choy and you have a great first-trimester dish.

SERVES 2

Prep time: 10 minutes
Cook time: 15 minutes

Ingredients

4–6 slices of very firm tofu, cut into bite-size cubes
400ml/13½fl oz/1¾ cups vegetable stock
5cm/1in piece of fresh root ginger, peeled and finely chopped
1 red chilli, deseeded and finely chopped
2 lemongrass stalks, chopped
2 limes
1 carrot, sliced
6–8 chestnut/cremini mushrooms, sliced
1 x 400ml/14fl oz can of coconut milk
1 tablespoon fish sauce
2 tomatoes, quartered
16 king prawns/jumbo shrimp
1 pak choi/bok choy, sliced
A few coriander/cilantro sprigs, leaves chopped

1 Preheat the oven to 180°C/350°F/Gas 4.

2 Place the tofu on a baking sheet and bake for 15 minutes.

3 Pour the stock into a saucepan over a medium heat and bring to the boil. Add the ginger, chilli and lemongrass along with the juice of 1 of the limes. Reduce the heat to low and keep at a simmer.

4 Add the carrot and mushrooms, then pour in the coconut milk and fish sauce. Bring back to the boil before reducing to a simmer.

5 Add the tomatoes and cook for another 5 minutes. Add the prawns/shrimp and pak choi/bok choy and cook for another 2 minutes until the prawns turn pink. Squeeze in the juice of the remaining lime. Add the tofu and chopped coriander/cilantro before serving.

>> **MIX IT UP:**
* Swap the tofu and prawns/shrimp for chicken or beef, or leave out the prawns for a vegan option.
* Add whole-wheat noodles for some carbs.

Harissa-Roasted Butterfly Chicken with Olive & Tomato Couscous & Parsley Mint Yogurt

A smoky dish that's perfect for those evenings when all mum-to-be wants to do is curl up on the couch with a good meal. The parsley and mint yogurt adds a zing while adding calcium and folate.

SERVES 2
Prep time: 15 minutes
Cook time: 25 minutes

Ingredients

2 chicken breasts
2 teaspoons harissa paste (or tomato
   purée for a spice-free option)
Juice of 1 lemon
12 cherry tomatoes
2 tablespoons olive oil
1 onion, diced
60g/2¼oz/½ cup pitted green olives
600ml/21fl oz/2½ cups chicken stock
250g/9oz/1⅔ cups couscous
Knob of butter
1 garlic clove, finely chopped
a few mint sprigs, finely chopped
a few parsley sprigs, finely chopped
6 tablespoons Greek yogurt (or a
   plant-based alternative)
Salt

> **>> MIX IT UP:**
> * Roast cauliflower steaks instead of chicken breasts.
> * Swap the couscous for brown rice, mashed sweet potato, or quinoa.
> * Sprinkle pomegranate seeds for extra nutrients.

1 Preheat the oven to 180°C/350°F/Gas 4.

2 Using a sharp knife butterfly the chicken breasts by cutting them in half width-wise (make sure you don't cut all the way through) and open them up like a book. Rub the harissa paste into the chicken along with a pinch of salt, place the breasts on a baking sheet, squeeze over the lemon and roast for 25 minutes. Remove when cooked and keep warm.

3 Place the cherry tomatoes in a baking pan, sprinkle with some salt, drizzle over a tablespoon of olive oil and roast alongside the chicken for 25 minutes.

4 Heat another tablespoon of oil in a saucepan over a medium heat. Add the onion and cook for a few minutes. Add the sliced olives and cook for a further 2 minutes. Add the chicken stock to the pan and bring to the boil, then remove from the heat, add the couscous and cover with a lid. Leave for 10 minutes, then stir in the knob of butter and fluff with a fork.

5 Combine the garlic, parsley and mint with the yogurt in a bowl.

6 Remove the tomatoes from the oven and mix into the couscous. Divide between 2 plates and place the chicken on top. And the parsley and mint yogurt before serving.

Coconut Black Rice Pudding & Cinnamon Bananas Topped with Coconut Caramel

Oh, just where to start with this dish! Rich and creamy coconut black rice, sweet bananas and rich vegan coconut caramel drizzled over the top. A truly delicious dessert that is packed full of antioxidants and fibre and also gives mum-to-be a load of nutrients suitable for the first trimester. The caramel will last up to a week in the fridge.

SERVES 2
Prep time: 5 minutes
Cook time: 45 minutes

✳ VEGETARIAN
✳ FAMILY-FRIENDLY

Ingredients

250g/9oz/1 cup black rice
400ml/14fl oz/1⅔ cups cold water
2 x 400ml/14fl oz cans of coconut milk
2 tablespoons chia seeds
8–10 tablespoons maple syrup
a knob of butter
1 teaspoon of cinnamon
2 bananas, sliced at an angle
Salt

>> **MIX IT UP:**
✳ Other vitamin-rich fruits work well here, such as mango, papaya or orange.
✳ Other seeds, such as flaxseeds or sunflower seeds, would also work well instead of the chia.

1 Place the black rice in a pan and add 400ml/14fl oz/1⅔ cups cold water. Bring to the boil, then add 1 can of the coconut milk. Bring it back to the boil, then reduce to a simmer. Cook uncovered for 20 minutes, then cover and cook for another 20 minutes. Remove from the heat, stir in the chia seeds and keep covered.

2 Pour the other can of coconut milk into a separate pan, add the maple syrup and bring to the boil. Reduce to a simmer for around 20 minutes until the volume of liquid has halved. Remove from the heat and leave to cool and refrigerate until needed.

3 Melt the butter in a frying pan over a medium heat. Sprinkle the cinnamon over the bananas along with a pinch of salt and cook for a few minutes, turning once until they begin to colour.

4 Divide the rice between 2 bowls, place some banana slices on top of each and drizzle with the coconut caramel.

Pomegranate & Raspberry Chocolate Bites

If mum-to-be is craving chocolate in the first trimester, give these a whirl. They're a great treat to make and each bite contains a juicy burst of vitamin C from the pomegranate. I love this recipe as it takes only 5 minutes and works with so many different fruits. You will need an empty ice cube tray. Bookmark this recipe for a great snack while doing late-night feeds when baby arrives!

MAKES 8

Prep time: 10 minutes, plus 2 hours freezing time

✻ BATCH-COOK ME!

Ingredients

200g/7oz good-quality chocolate

50g/1¾oz/¼ cup pomegranate seeds

50g/1¾oz/⅓ cup raspberries

1 Place a large heatproof bowl over a pan of gently simmering water, making sure the bowl doesn't touch the water. Break the chocolate up into small pieces and place in the bowl, allowing the heat from below to slowly melt it.

2 Half fill each compartment of the ice-cube tray with the melted chocolate. Spoon a few pomegranate seeds or half a raspberry into each one, then fill with the remaining chocolate. Place in the freezer for at least 2 hours.

3 Remove the chocolate from the tray and using a sharp knife cut the cubes in half. Use any remaining fruit to sprinkle over the chocolate. Eat immediately before they begin to melt.

>> **MIX IT UP:**
✻ Endless possibilities here. Go for milk or white chocolate (but I think the darker the better).
✻ Experiment with different fruits like passionfruit, blueberries, strawberries, orange and pear.

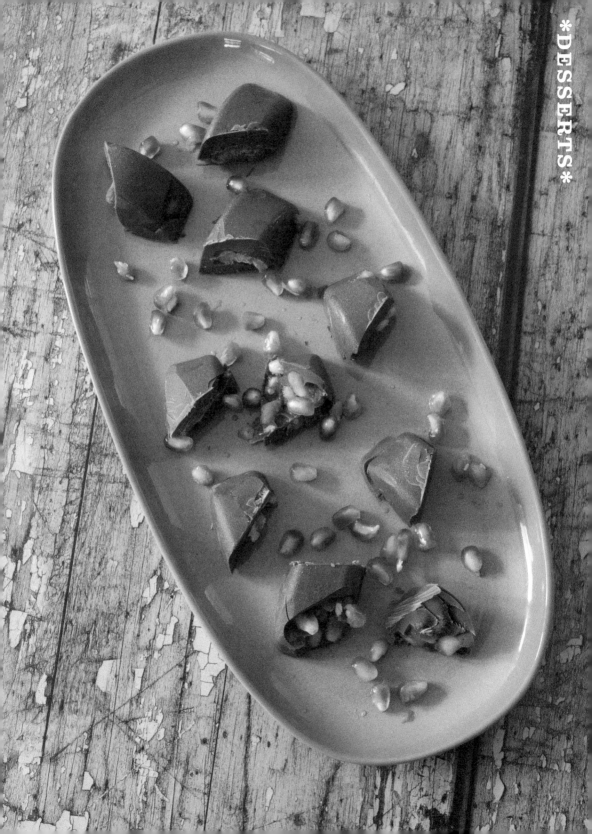

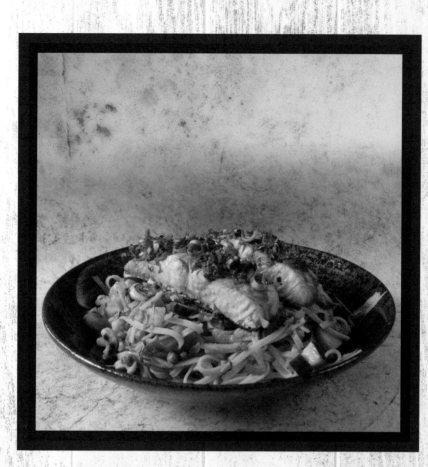

CHAPTER 2:

The Honeymoon
Trimester
(weeks 13−26)

Eating Well in the Honeymoon Trimester

Ah, the second trimester, also known as the honeymoon trimester as it's a time when, hopefully, mum-to-be is beginning to feel more like herself again. Any morning sickness has likely passed, her energy is beginning to return and, if the pregnancy has been a secret up until now, she's maybe beginning to share the good news with the world! With all these changes, non-beige food is beginning to become appealing again, and so the second trimester is the time to eat the rainbow. Vegetables and fruits that may have been shunned for the last 12 weeks are now getting interesting again, some strong-smelling foods, such as fish, are now back in play and, in general, mum-to-be may be more open to eating a wider variety of foods. Embrace and enjoy this time!

The fog clears and the appetite returns

If the first trimester was all about creating life, the second trimester is all about growing that life. Again, it's important to say that as long as mum-to-be is taking her recommended vitamin supplements, there is nothing specific that absolutely has to be eaten; however, there are certain types of foods high in various nutrients that are great for mum-to-be and baby during the second trimester. As well as continuing to eat a balanced diet, it's a good idea to eat foods that contain omega-3 for baby's brain development and foods that contain vitamin D for strong bone and teeth development. Iron is also important, as it helps stimulate red blood cell growth – in pregnancy a woman is carrying 50 per cent more blood than usual, so iron-rich foods are a real help.

In general, if mum-to-be is feeling good about food and her appetite has returned, try to incorporate extra nutrient-rich ingredients into your meals, even if it's something simple like adding frozen peas to a bowl of pasta or lentils to a salad.

Try to build in two portions of fish per week (or other foods rich in omega-3, see next page). Also try to incorporate a variety of bright, colourful fruit and vegetables into mealtimes. Now is the time to eat the rainbow! You could add fruit, veg, nuts and seeds to rice dishes, eat lots of tasty salads, vegetable- and fruit-packed stir-fries, chilled soups and so on.

What to focus on

>> **OMEGA-3-RICH FOODS**: Oily fish such as salmon, trout and mackerel contain, amongst other good stuff, lots of omega-3. Non-fish sources of omega-3 include walnuts, pumpkin seeds, linseeds/flaxseeds and chia seeds.

>> **EAT THE RAINBOW**: In general, the brighter the fruit and veg, the more nutrients it contains, so go for lots of peppers, chillies, carrots, avocados, broccoli, berries, oranges and mangos.

>> **VITAMIN D**: Mushrooms can be good sources of vitamin D. Salmon and trout, egg yolks, butter and cheese also contain vitamin D.

>> **IRON**: Red meats, shellfish, beans, pulses/legumes, nuts and dried fruits are all good sources of iron.

In this chapter you'll find lots of recipes featuring omega-3-rich foods, vibrant fruit and vegetables packed full of nutrients and ideas for easily increasing iron intake.

SPOTLIGHT:

Five Easy, Healthy & Colourful Salads to Embrace the Honeymoon Trimester

Salads may have been totally off the menu in the first trimester but now they're back with a bang. Fruit and vegetables don't need to be hidden during this phase; they can now take centre stage as mum-to-be's appetite – in most cases – returns to what it was previously.

Not only are salads quick, they're also full of brilliantly healthy foods and can be made from pretty much any fruit and veg you have to hand. Salads combine lots of different food sources, so whatever salad you choose always think about what extra nutrients you can add; try cheeses, nuts, seeds, pulses/legumes and herbs.

Halloumi, Mango, Avocado & Cucumber Salad with a Lemon & Thyme Dressing

SERVES 2
Prep time: 10 minutes
Cook time: 7 minutes

✳ VEGETARIAN

Ingredients

3 tablespoons olive oil ✳ 200g/7oz halloumi, sliced ✳ ½ cucumber, diced ✳ 1 avocado, peeled, destoned and diced ✳ 1 lemon ✳ 1 large mango, diced ✳ A few thyme sprigs, leaves picked, or 1 tablespoon dried thyme

1 Heat a tablespoon of oil in a frying pan over a medium heat. Add the halloumi and cook for around 7 minutes, turning once. Set aside.

2 Dice the cucumber and avocado. Squeeze half the lemon over. Place in a bowl and add the mango.

3 In a small bowl or jug mix together 2 tablespoons of the oil, the juice from the other half of the lemon and the thyme.

4 Tear the halloumi into small pieces and mix into the salad. Drizzle over the dressing and serve.

Halloumi, Lentil & Pomegranate Salad with a Miso Dressing

SERVES 2
Prep time: 10 minutes
Cook time: 7 minutes

✳ VEGETARIAN

Ingredients

1 teaspoon olive oil ✳ 200g/7oz (roughly 1 pack) halloumi, sliced ✳ ½ a cucumber, diced ✳ 1 shallot, diced ✳ 1 x 400g/14oz can of green lentils, drained ✳ 50g/1¾oz/½ cup almonds ✳ 4 tablespoons pomegranate seeds ✳ A handful of rocket/arugula ✳ 1 avocado, peeled, destoned and diced ✳ 3 tablespoons sesame oil ✳ 1 tablespoon miso paste ✳ 1 teaspoon rice wine or red wine vinegar ✳ 1 teaspoon honey ✳ 1 teaspoon lemon juice

1 Heat the olive oil in a frying pan over a medium heat. Add the halloumi and cook for around 7 minutes, turning once. Set aside to cool.

2 Place the cucumber and shallot in a bowl along with the lentils, almonds, pomegranate seeds, rocket/arugula and avocado.

3 Mix the sesame oil, miso, vinegar, honey and lemon juice together well, then drizzle over the salad.

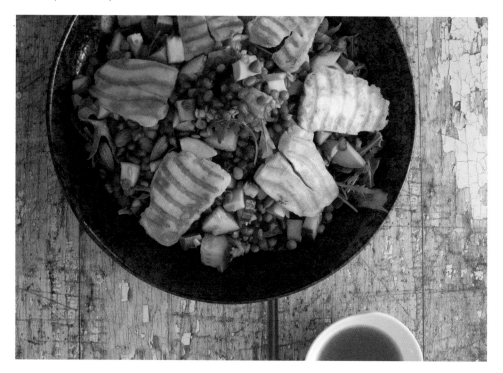

Roasted Fig, Feta & Walnut Salad with Orange, Avocado & Toasted Pumpkin Seeds

SERVES 2
Prep time: 10 minutes
Cook time: 10 minutes

✱ VEGETARIAN

Ingredients

A handful of walnuts ✱ 2 teaspoons pumpkin seeds ✱ 6–8 figs ✱ 100g/3½oz/½ cup crumbled feta cheese (or mozzarella if you prefer) ✱ 2 handfuls of rocket/arugula ✱ 2 handfuls of spinach leaves, chopped ✱ 2 oranges, separated into segments ✱ 2 avocados, peeled, destoned and diced ✱ ½ cucumber, diced ✱ Juice of 1 lemon ✱ Olive oil, for drizzling ✱ 2 teaspoons honey ✱ Salt and black pepper

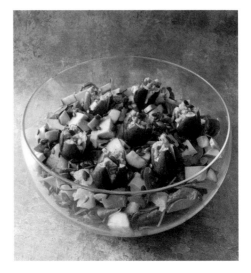

1 Preheat the oven to 160°C/315°F/Gas 3.

2 In a hot frying pan over a medium heat, dry fry the walnuts and pumpkin seeds for 3 minutes. Leave to cool and then crush the walnuts.

3 Slice the figs in a criss-cross to about two-thirds of the way down. Gently pull them apart and fill with the crumbled feta. Place on a baking sheet and bake for 5–7 minutes until the feta begins to melt.

4 Meanwhile, mix the rocket/arugula and spinach leaves in a bowl and add the orange segments, avocado and cucumber. Lightly season, squeeze over the lemon juice and drizzle with olive oil.

5 Remove the figs from the oven and drizzle the honey over them. Place the figs in the salad bowl and sprinkle over the toasted pumpkin seeds and walnuts. Serve while the figs are still warm.

Orzo & Salmon Salad with a Salsa Verde Dressing

SERVES 2
Prep time: 15 minutes
Cook time: 10 minutes

Ingredients

200g/7oz/1 cup orzo ✳ 1 lemon ✳ 2 salmon fillets, about 150g/5½oz each, skin on ✳ 1 shallot, diced ✳ 12 cherry tomatoes, halved ✳ 1 red pepper, cored, deseeded and diced ✳ 1 avocado, peeled, destoned and diced ✳ ½ cucumber, diced ✳ 80g/3oz pitted black or green olives ✳ 1 garlic clove ✳ a bunch of parsley, roughly chopped ✳ 1 teaspoon white wine vinegar ✳ 3–4 tablespoons olive oil ✳ Salt

1 Heat the oven to 180°C/350°F/Gas 4.

2 Cook the orzo as per the packet instructions, then drain and cool.

3 Finely grate the lemon zest and set aside in a small bowl. Cut 4 slices from the lemon and arrange on a baking sheet. Place the salmon fillets on top and bake for 10 minutes, then remove, leave to cool and flake into chunks. Discard the skin.

4 Mix together the shallot, cherry tomatoes, red pepper, avocado, cucumber and olives in a salad bowl.

5 To make the salsa verde, place the lemon zest, garlic, parsley, white wine vinegar and olive oil in a food processor. Squeeze in the juice from the remaining piece of lemon, add a pinch of salt and blend together. Add more olive oil for a thinner dressing.

6 Add the cooled orzo to the salad bowl and mix well. Top with the flaked cooked salmon and drizzle over the salsa verde before serving.

>> **MIX IT UP:**
✳ Traditional salsa verde also includes capers and anchovies but they can be a strong taste for pregnancy, so I've left them out. You could add them in, if you prefer.
✳ For a vegan option, cauliflower steaks instead of the salmon are delicious with a salsa verde.

Greek Salad with Rosemary & Lemon Grilled Chicken

SERVES 2
Prep time: 10 minutes
Cook time: 15 minutes

Ingredients

5 tablespoons olive oil ✳ 1 chicken breast, cut into 5 or 6 pieces ✳ 1 lemon ✳ A few rosemary sprigs, leaves picked, or 1 tablespoon dried rosemary ✳ 8 large vine tomatoes, quartered (or cut into 6 if they're large) ✳ 1 red onion, diced ✳ 1 large cucumber, diced ✳ 100g/3½oz/ generous 1 cup pitted black olives ✳ 2 avocados, peeled and destoned ✳ 100g/3½oz feta cheese (or a plant-based alternative) ✳ 1 teaspoon finely chopped oregano or 1 teaspoon dried ✳ Salt

1 Heat a tablespoon of the oil in a frying pan over a medium heat. Add the chicken breast to the pan. Squeeze over the juice of half the lemon, sprinkle over the rosemary and cook for 15 minutes, turning once.

2 Meanwhile, assemble the salad. Place the tomatoes and onion in a bowl along with a generous pinch of salt.

3 Add the cucumber and olives.

4 Dice the avocados, squeeze over the juice from the other half of the lemon to stop them going brown, then add to the bowl.

5 Crumble over the feta, sprinkle over the oregano and add the remaining olive oil. Mix well. Either top with the cooked chicken or serve it on the side.

> > **MIX IT UP:**
✳ The chicken is completely optional, so leave it out, if you prefer.
✳ Or you could swap it for some roasted white fish (roast it with rosemary and oregano).
✳ Swap the feta for vegan feta or tofu.

Green Shakshuka

Instead of a traditional shakshuka, try this version, which is full to the brim with wonderful greens, herbs and chillies. This is a great weekend brunch dish for mum-to-be to enjoy, safe in the knowledge that she's getting a big dose of folate and other vitamins, iron and fibre. Plus, it's on the table in 20 minutes!

SERVES 2–3
Prep time: 5 minutes
Cook time: 15 minutes

✳ VEGETARIAN
✳ FAMILY-FRIENDLY

Ingredients

A knob of butter (or a plant-based
    alternative)
1 shallot, diced
1 garlic clove
1 green chilli
1 teaspoon ground cumin
1 teaspoon ground coriander
Around 5 handfuls of spinach leaves,
    chopped
100g/3½oz/1½ cups kale or cavolo
    nero, tough stalks removed, roughly
    chopped
4–6 eggs
1 teaspoon harissa paste (optional)
A few coriander/cilantro sprigs, leaves
    chopped
A few parsley sprigs, leaves chopped

1 Melt the butter in a frying pan over a medium heat. Add the shallot and cook for 2–3 minutes. Then add the garlic and chilli to the pan along with the ground cumin and ground coriander. Mix well and cook for another 2–3 minutes.

2 Add the spinach and kale to the pan and cook for a few minutes until wilted.

3 Make spaces in the greens and crack in the eggs. Cover the pan and cook for 3–4 minutes.

4 Remove the pan from the heat. Dot the harissa over the eggs, if using, then sprinkle over the fresh coriander/cilantro and parsley.

> > **MIX IT UP:**
✳ Add in other greens, such as peas, leeks or courgettes/zucchini.
✳ Dice up some bacon or chorizo and cook in the pan before adding the spinach and kale.
✳ Crumble over some feta.

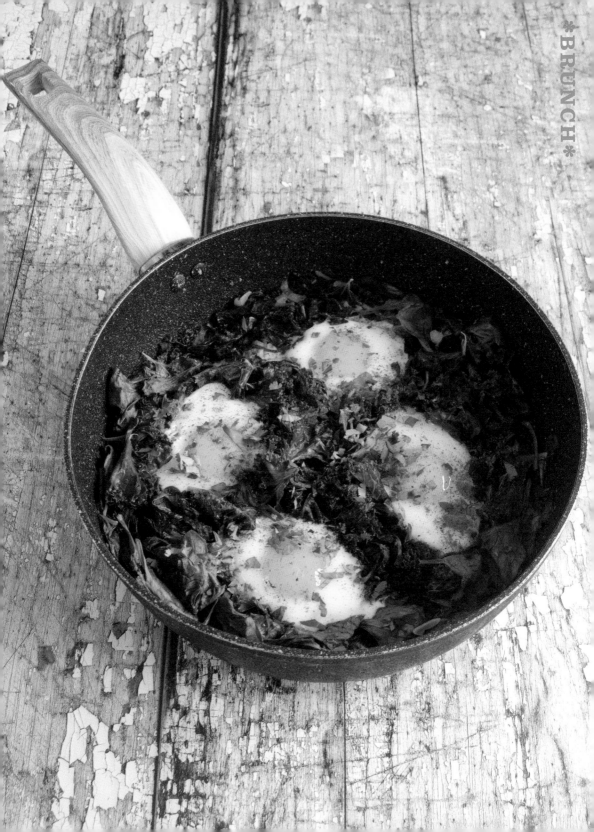

Three Chilled Soups Bursting with Flavour

These soups are all easy to make, refreshing and will give mum-to-be a real boost because of their high vegetable content. If the second trimester coincides with some warm weather, even better: make a bowl and enjoy in the sun.

* EACH RECIPE SERVES 2 *
* PREP TIME: 5–10 MINUTES *
* COOK TIME: UNDER 10 MINUTES *

Mango, Squash, Coconut and Green Chilli

Ingredients

200ml/7fl oz/scant 1 cup vegetable stock
1 green chilli
1 butternut squash, peeled and diced
200ml/7fl oz/scant 1 cup coconut milk
2 mangoes, chopped
2 tablespoons desiccated coconut
2 tablespoons black sesame seeds

* VEGAN
* FAMILY-FRIENDLY, just leave out the chilli

>> **MIX IT UP:**
* Papaya would work well instead of mango.
* Roast the squash first for more depth of flavour.

METHOD

1 Pour the stock into a saucepan over a medium heat and bring to the boil. Add the chilli and butternut squash, bring back to the boil and cook 5 minutes.

2 Add the coconut milk. Stir in the mango and cook for a further 2–3 minutes.

3 Blend until smooth with a hand-held/immersion blender. Alternatively, transfer to a blender and blitz until smooth. Leave to cool, then refrigerate until required (maximum 48 hours).

4 In a hot dry frying pan over a medium heat, toast the desiccated coconut and sesame seeds for 2 minutes. Serve on top of the soup.

Thai Gazpacho

Ingredients

12 ripe tomatoes, chopped
1 red pepper, cored, deseeded and chopped
1 red chilli, diced
1 shallot, chopped
½ cucumber, chopped
Juice of 1 lime
3 tablespoons sesame oil
2 teaspoons fish sauce
2 teaspoons red wine vinegar
A few coriander/cilantro sprigs, leaves picked
A few mint sprigs, leaves picked

METHOD

1 Place the tomatoes, pepper and chilli in a blender. Reserve a teaspoon each of the shallot and cucumber and add the rest to the blender.

2 Add the lime juice, sesame oil, fish sauce and red wine vinegar. Reserve a few of the coriander/cilantro and mint leaves and add the rest to the blender. Blitz until smooth.

3 Refrigerate until required but preferably within a few hours. When ready to serve, top with the reserved shallot, cucumber, coriander and mint.

Asparagus, Mint and Pea

Ingredients

600ml/20fl oz/2½ cups vegetable stock
200g/7oz/1 cup frozen peas
24 asparagus spears, woody ends removed, chopped
A few mint sprigs, leaves picked
Olive oil, to serve

✳ VEGAN
✳ FAMILY-FRIENDLY

METHOD

1 Pour the stock into a saucepan over a medium heat and bring to the boil. Add the peas and asparagus and cook for 5 minutes.

2 Remove from the heat, add most of the mint (reserving a few leaves) and blend until smooth with a hand-held/immersion blender.

3 Allow to cool, then refrigerate until required (maximum 48 hours). Sprinkle the remaining mint over the soup before serving.

>> **MIX IT UP:**
✳ Don't add the chilli if you don't want the spice.
✳ Keep it chunky and serve it as a sauce for chicken or prawns/shrimp.

>> **MIX IT UP:**
✳ Add some bacon or ham to the soup.
✳ Swap broccoli for asparagus, if you prefer.
✳ Grate some cheese over the top.

Anni's Favourite Pregnancy Smoothies

As mum-to-be's appetite for fruit and vegetables re-emerges, smoothies come back into play. They're a great way to increase not only folate intake but fibre and other nutrients too. My wife got back into smoothies in a big way first time round in her second trimester, and here are her three favourite recipes.

All of these recipes make a little over 300ml/10½fl oz/scant 1¼ cup, or 1 serving.

Green:
Perfect for a Folate Injection

Blend together a handful each of spinach and kale, 1 apple, the juice of 1 lemon, a 5cm/2in piece of fresh root ginger, ½ a banana and ½ a pear. Top up with 200ml/7fl oz/scant 1 cup coconut water, or to your chosen consistency.

Pink:
A Great Immune Booster

Blend together 2 carrots, the juice of 1 lemon and 1 orange, a 5cm/2in piece of fresh root ginger, 1 pre-cooked beetroot/beet and ½ teaspoon of ground turmeric. Top up with 200ml/7fl oz/scant 1 cup coconut water, or to your chosen consistency.

Purple:
A Nutritious Breakfast Smoothie

Blend together 1 banana, a handful of blueberries, 2 tablespoons of almonds and ½ teaspoon of ground cinnamon. Top up with 200ml/7fl oz/scant 1 cup coconut milk, or to your chosen consistency.

Lemongrass-Roasted Salmon with a Spicy Miso Noodle Salad «

This is pure second trimester on a plate. Omega-3-rich salmon infused with beautiful flavours alongside a vibrant noodle salad is everything mum-to-be needs at this time, and a delicious dish for whoever's eating. If it's warm outside, do this on the barbecue!

SERVES 2

Prep time: 15 minutes

Cook time: 12 minutes

Ingredients

3 teaspoons soy sauce

2 teaspoons sriracha or other hot sauce

2 teaspoons rice wine vinegar, or red wine vinegar

a bunch of coriander/cilantro, chopped

1 lemongrass stalk, finely chopped

5cm/2in piece of fresh root ginger, peeled and grated

2 garlic cloves, crushed

2 salmon fillets (around 200g/7oz each)

½ lime

200g/7oz whole-wheat noodles

small handful of cashew nuts

2 carrots, grated

½ cucumber, diced

1 red pepper, cored, deseeded and diced

1 shallot, diced

50g/1¾oz/¼ cup fresh or defrosted peas

1 tablespoon miso paste

3 tablespoons sesame oil

1 teaspoon honey

« Photo on page 48

1 Preheat the oven to 180°C/350°F/Gas 4. Line a baking pan with foil.

2 For the marinade, mix the soy sauce, 1 teaspoon of the sriracha and 1 teaspoon of the vinegar. Add the lemongrass, ginger and 1 garlic clove.

3 Place the salmon in the foil-lined baking pan and pour over the marinade. If you have time, cover and refrigerate for an hour or so. If not, don't worry. Squeeze over the lime juice, then bake for 12 minutes. Remove from the oven, then garnish with the coriander.

4 Meanwhile, cook the noodles as per the packet instructions. Drain and leave to cool. Cook the cashew nuts in a dry pan for 2−3 minutes and then set aside.

5 Next, make the salad. Place the carrot, cucumber, red pepper and shallot in a bowl. Add the peas, cashew nuts and noodles. Mix well.

6 For the salad dressing, combine the miso, sesame oil, honey, remaining sriracha, vinegar and garlic in a bowl. Pour over the salad, mix and serve with the salmon.

> > **MIX IT UP:**
> * The marinade works well with tuna, tofu, mushrooms, prawns or chicken thighs.
> * Leave out the noodles and add cooked broccoli for a lighter salad.

Grilled Japanese Mackerel, Cucumber, Soba Noodles and Miso Soup

In Japan, grilled mackerel is a frequently eaten morning dish, so I wanted to include it here in the brunch section, especially because mackerel is such a good fish to eat in the second trimester. I love the combination of the smoky mackerel, salty miso, sweet cucumber and chewy soba noodles. The tofu and soba noodles are great sources of protein, while seaweed contains omega-3 and folate as well as other nutrients.

SERVES 2
Prep time: 15 minutes
Cook time: 5 minutes

✳ FAMILY-FRIENDLY

Ingredients

3 tablespoons soy sauce

1 teaspoon rice wine vinegar or white wine vinegar

1 teaspoon sesame oil

1 garlic clove, crushed

5cm/2in piece of fresh root ginger, peeled and finely grated

2 tablespoons olive oil

2 smoked mackerel fillets, about 180g /6¼oz each, skin on

10cm/4in piece of cucumber, sliced lengthways

200g/7oz of soba noodles

2 sheets of nori seaweed, cut into strips

2 spring onions/scallions, thinly sliced

100g/3½oz firm tofu, diced

2 tablespoons miso paste

1 First, make the marinade. In a bowl combine the soy sauce, rice wine vinegar and sesame oil. Add the garlic and ginger.

2 Heat the olive oil in a pan over a medium heat. Add the mackerel fillets, spoon over half the marinade and fry skin-side down for 2–3 minutes. As the mackerel fillets are already cooked, we are just warming them up.

3 Place the cucumber slices on a plate and spoon over the remaining marinade.

4 Cook the soba noodles as per the packet instructions. Drain and divide between 2 bowls.

5 Divide the seaweed, spring onions/ scallions and tofu between two bowls, add a spoonful of miso paste to each bowl and half-fill with boiling water.

> > **MIX IT UP:**
> ✳ Add some chilli or hot sauce to the marinade for more heat.
> ✳ Swap the mackerel for salmon.

Salmon Steak with Black Rice and Mango and Chilli Salsa, Charred Spring Onion, Coriander Sweetcorn

This is my favourite recipe in the book and one I've made many a time for my wife, both during pregnancy and not. The salmon has a lovely smokiness from the spices, which goes so well with the fresh mango salsa. Black rice is such a good source of nutrients and the addition of coriander/cilantro and sweetcorn is a really easy way of getting more vitamins in. I hope you love it as much as my family does.

SERVES 2
Prep time: 10 minutes
Cook time: 25 minutes

Ingredients
250g/9oz/1½ cups black rice
1 mango, diced
½ red chilli, deseeded and diced
1 shallot, diced
1 tomato, diced
A few coriander/cilantro sprigs, leaves chopped
1 tablespoon red wine vinegar
1 lime
1 teaspoon ground cumin
1 teaspoon paprika
2 salmon steaks, about 150g/5½oz each
200g/7oz/1 cup frozen sweetcorn
2 teaspoons olive oil
6–8 spring onions/scallions
Salt

> > **MIX IT UP:**
> * Try trout, chicken or pork instead of salmon.
> * Use brown rice or noodles.

1 Preheat the oven to 180°C/350°F/Gas 4.

2 Cook the rice as per the packet instructions; it will take around 25 minutes.

3 Meanwhile, make the salsa. In a bowl, mix together the mango, chilli, shallot, tomato and most of the coriander/cilantro. Spoon over the vinegar and the juice of half the lime. Mix well, add a pinch of salt and refrigerate until needed.

4 Spoon the cumin and paprika onto a plate and mix with the juice of the other half lime. Lay the salmon on top and rub the spices in. Place the salmon on a baking tray and cook in the oven for 10–12 minutes.

5 Place the sweetcorn in a bowl and pour over boiling water to defrost. Drain, leave to cool slightly, then add the reserved coriander.

6 Heat a teaspoon of the oil in a griddle/grill pan over a high heat. Add the spring onions/scallions with a pinch of salt and cook for a few minutes on each side. Remove and set aside.

7 Divide the rice between 2 plates and top with the spring onion, salmon and salsa. Serve with the sweetcorn alongside.

Fruit Stir-fries

Cooking with fruit doesn't just increase the vitamin content of a dish, it also adds loads of flavour. The sweetness of fruit balances a spicy, salty stir-fry wonderfully; my favourite is the combination of prawns, mango and chilli. Serve with wholegrain rice, noodles or lettuce cups.

✳ BATCH-COOK ME! ✳

Prawn, Mango and Chilli

SERVES 2
Prep time: 10 minutes
Cook time: 10 minutes

Ingredients

3 tablespoons soy sauce

1 teaspoon sriracha or an alternative hot sauce

1 teaspoon honey

2 tablespoons sesame oil

5cm/2in piece of fresh root ginger, peeled
and grated

200g/7oz raw peeled prawns/shrimp

1 onion, diced

1 red chilli, deseeded and diced

1 green pepper, cored, deseeded and sliced

1 courgette/zucchini, sliced

2 mangos, diced

1 head of pak choi/bok choy, sliced

A few coriander/cilantro leaves

METHOD

1 In a bowl, combine the soy sauce, sriracha, honey and 1 tablespoon of the sesame oil. Add the ginger and prawns/shrimp and mix well.

2 Heat the remaining sesame oil in a frying pan over a medium heat. Add the onion and cook for 3 minutes. Add the chilli, green pepper and courgette. Cook for 2 minutes.

3 Add the mango, pour in the prawns and sauce, then cook for a further 2 minutes.

4 Finally, add the pak choi/bok choy and cook for another minute. Serve sprinkled with coriander/cilantro.

> >> **MIX IT UP:**
> ✳ Chicken would work well instead of or alongside the prawns/shrimp.
> ✳ Grate some carrot into the pan or add a few broccoli florets, both of which would complement the mango.

Beef, Orange and Cashew Nut

SERVES 2

Prep time: 10 minutes
Cook time: 10 minutes

Ingredients

3 large oranges

4 tablespoons soy sauce

1 teaspoon cornflour/cornstarch

1 teaspoon rice wine vinegar, or red wine vinegar

1 garlic clove, crushed

5cm/2in piece of fresh root ginger, peeled
   and grated

1 sirloin or rump steak, about 200g/7oz, cubed

2 tablespoons cashew nuts

1 tablespoon sesame oil

1 shallot, diced

1 red pepper, cored, deseeded and diced

1 carrot, diced

1 courgette/zucchini, diced

1 head of pak choi/bok choy, sliced

METHOD

1 Peel the oranges, cut 2½ of them into segments and set aside.

2 To make the marinade, squeeze the juice from the remaining orange half into a bowl. Add the soy sauce, cornflour, vinegar, garlic and ginger. Place the beef in the bowl, ensuring it's covered by the marinade.

3 In a hot frying pan over a high heat, dry-fry the cashew nuts for 2 minutes until toasted, then set aside.

4 Heat the sesame oil in a frying pan over a high heat. Add the shallot, then the red pepper, carrot and courgette/zucchini and cook for 2–3 minutes. Add the beef and marinade to the pan and cook for a further 3–4 minutes. Finally, add the pak choi/bok choy and cook for a further minute before serving.

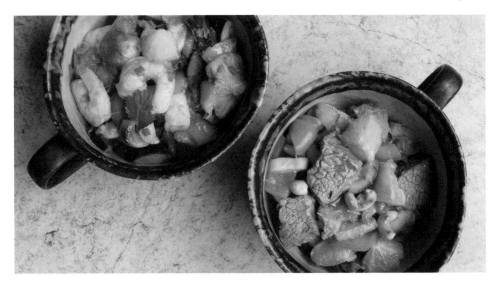

Tahini and Paprika-Roasted Chicken Thighs with Pomegranate, Mint and Pistachio Rice

Mint and pomegranate enhance the flavour of rice and add texture, making each spoonful that much more enjoyable. The chicken has a little heat from the paprika, matching well with the yogurt. A top dish full of everything mum-to-be needs in the second trimester.

SERVES 2–3
Prep time: 10 minutes
Cook time: 25 minutes

* FAMILY-FRIENDLY, as long as there are no nut allergies

Ingredients

8–9 chicken thighs skin-on (either bone-in or deboned)
3 tablespoons tahini
1 tablespoon paprika
1 tablespoon olive oil
250g/9oz/1¼ cups brown basmati rice
50g/1¾oz/⅓ cup shelled pistachio nuts, crushed
Seeds from ½ pomegranate
A few mint sprigs, leaves chopped
3 tablespoons Greek yogurt (or a plant-based alternative)
Salt

> > **MIX IT UP:**
> * Stir a few pulses/ legumes through the rice or add in some diced cucumber and carrots.
> * Use the same marinade to cook a head of cauliflower or broccoli.

1 Preheat the oven to 180°C/350°F/Gas 4.

2 Place the chicken thighs in an ovenproof dish. In a bowl, mix together the tahini, paprika and olive oil, then spread over the chicken thighs, ensuring they're well covered. Season each thigh with a pinch of salt and roast for 20–25 minutes (if the bones are in they will take longer to cook).

3 Meanwhile, cook the rice as per the packet instructions, then drain and set aside to cool. Once cool, stir in the pistachios and pomegranate seeds, reserving 1 tablespoon of each. Add half the mint and mix well.

4 Remove the chicken from the oven and rest for 5 minutes.

5 Spoon the yogurt into a bowl and add half the reserved crushed pistachios, pomegranate and fresh mint.

6 Divide the rice between the plates, top with the chicken thighs, then sprinkle with the remaining pistachios, pomegranate and mint. Serve with the yogurt on the side.

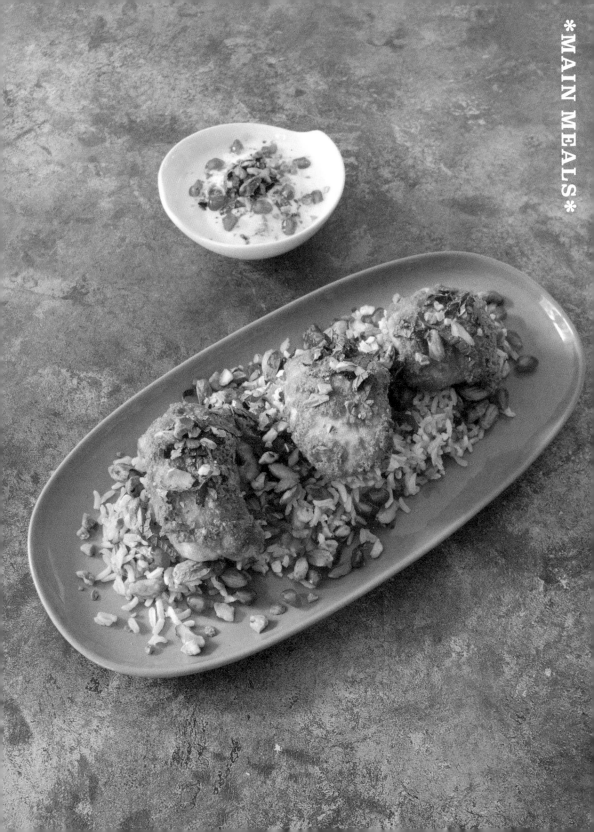

>> **MIX IT UP:**
* Prawns/shrimp would
work well instead of beef.
* Alternatively swap for
some roasted cauliflower
and broccoli.

Crunchy, Spicy Thai Beef Salad

In my opinion there's nothing tastier than a Thai beef salad. This dish is a gorgeous combination of crunchy vegetables, whole-wheat noodles, protein-rich beef and some spice, to make a filling and satisfying meal. Whenever I think of eating the rainbow, I think of this dish, so if mum-to-be's appetite has returned in the second trimester, get this on the menu.

SERVES 2

Prep time: 15 minutes

Cook time: 20 minutes

Ingredients

2–3 tablespoons of cashew nuts

Approx 200g/7oz whole-wheat noodles

1 lemongrass stalk, very thinly sliced

1 teaspoon brown sugar

Juice of 1 lime

2 teaspoons fish sauce

2 teaspoons sesame oil

1 red chilli, deseeded and finely diced

1 garlic clove, crushed

5cm/2in piece of fresh root ginger, peeled and finely grated

A bunch of coriander/cilantro, leaves chopped

1 sirloin or rump steak, about 200g/7oz

½ cucumber, sliced

2–3 carrots, sliced

2–3 spring onions/scallions, thinly sliced

A handful of cherry tomatoes, halved

A bunch of mint, leaves chopped

1 In a hot frying pan over a medium heat, dry-fry the cashew nuts for about 2–3 minutes until toasted, then set aside.

2 Cook the noodles as per packet instructions then drain and set aside.

3 Next make your dressing. Place the lemongrass in a bowl with the brown sugar, lime juice, fish sauce and sesame oil. Add the chilli, garlic, ginger and a few coriander/cilantro leaves and mix everything together well.

4 Cook the beef to your preference (2 minutes each side for medium-rare, 3 for medium and 4 for well done), then leave to rest for 10 minutes.

5 While the beef is resting, combine the cucumber, carrots, spring onions/scallions and tomatoes together in a salad bowl along with the cashew nuts, mint and remaining coriander. Pour over most of the dressing, reserving a teaspoon or two, and toss well.

6 Slice the beef into strips and place on top of the salad. Spoon over the remaining dressing before serving.

King Prawn and Pea Risotto with Coconut Milk and Turmeric

Risottos don't have to be just Italian-themed dishes; many non-European flavours and spices work well too. Here the creamy coconut-flavoured rice tastes great with the sweet bite of the prawns/shrimp and I love the colour the turmeric gives everything. Prawns are pure protein and a fantastic food for pregnancy. See page 178 for how to make arancini from leftover risotto.

SERVES 2, plus some
for the freezer
Prep time: 5 minutes
Cook time: 30 minutes

✳ BATCH-COOK ME!
✳ FAMILY FRIENDLY

Ingredients

A knob of butter (or a plant-based
alternative)
1 onion, diced
2 tablespoons ground turmeric
250g/9oz/1 cup Arborio rice
400ml/14fl oz/1⅔ cups fish stock
1 x 400ml/14fl oz can of coconut milk
100g/3½oz/½ cup frozen peas
12–16 raw peeled king prawns/
jumbo shrimp

1 Melt the butter in a pan over a medium heat. Add the onion and a tablespoon of turmeric and stir well. Cook for 2–3 minutes, then add the rice and stir well to ensure the onion and turmeric mixture coat the rice.

2 Add a ladleful of the stock and stir well. Keep stirring until most of the stock has been absorbed, then add another ladleful and repeat until all the stock has been used up (this will take around 20 minutes or so). While adding the stock, stir in the coconut milk, a little at a time, reserving 2 tablespoons for the prawns/shrimp.

3 When the rice is almost cooked, stir in the frozen peas. Remove the risotto from the heat and keep warm.

4 In a separate pan, mix the remaining tablespoon of turmeric with the reserved 2 tablespoons of coconut milk. Add the prawns and cook for about 3 minutes until pink.

5 Serve the risotto with the prawns on top.

> > **MIX IT UP:**
✳ Flaked salmon would work well instead of the prawns/shrimp, as would tofu.

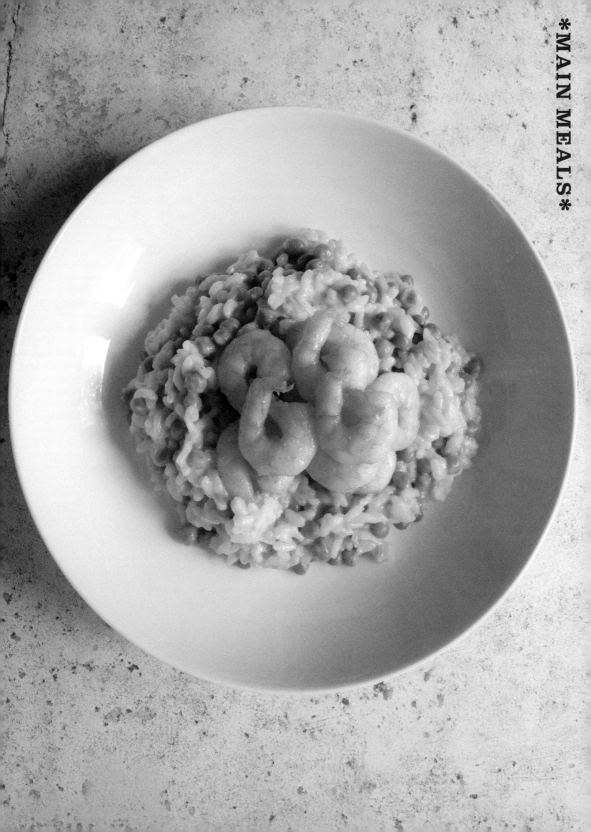

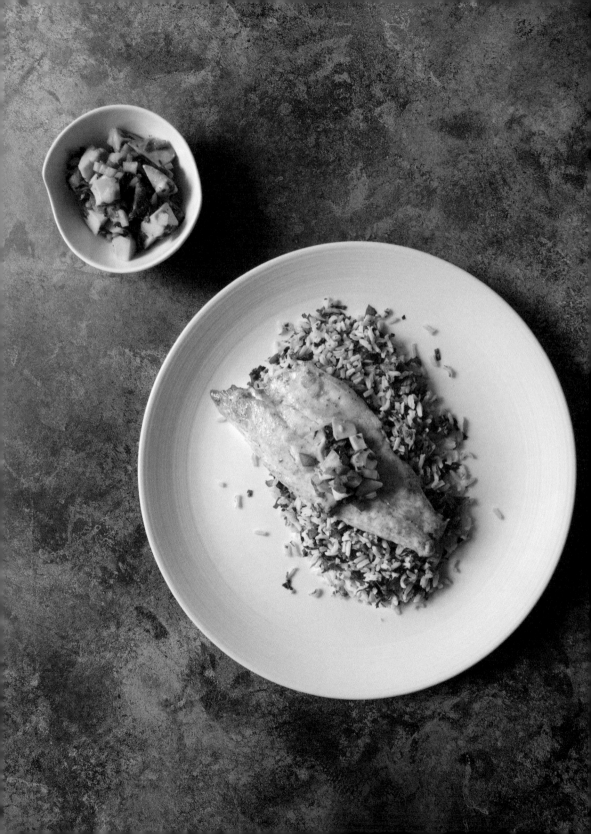

Pan-Fried Sea Bass with Coriander Rice and Avocado Salsa

Not only is sea bass great for mum-to-be nutritionally, but it only takes a couple of minutes to cook, so this makes a perfect midweek dish. The sweet, buttery fish combines really well with the sharp avocado salsa. It's delicious and a really fun dish to make.

SERVES 2

Prep time: 10 minutes

Cook time: 15 minutes

❊ FAMILY FRIENDLY without the salsa

Ingredients

250g/9oz/1¼ cups brown rice

½ avocado, peeled, destoned and diced

1 shallot, diced

1 red chilli, deseeded and diced

1 teaspoon red wine vinegar

A bunch of coriander/cilantro, leaves chopped

2 seabass fillets, about 150g/5½oz each, skin on

A knob of butter (or a plant-based alternative)

Salt and pepper

1 Cook the rice as per the packet instructions. Drain and keep warm.

2 Meanwhile, make the avocado salsa by mixing the avocado, shallot and chilli in a bowl with the red wine vinegar and a few chopped coriander/cilantro leaves. Refrigerate until needed.

3 Season the sea bass fillets. Melt the butter in a frying pan over a medium heat. Add the sea bass skin-side up and cook for 2 minutes, then gently flip over and cook for another 2 minutes, basting the fish with the butter. Remove and set aside.

4 Stir the remaining coriander through the rice. Serve alongside the sea bass topped with the avocado salsa.

>> **MIX IT UP:**

❊ This dish works well in a wrap.

❊ Serve with slices of avocado instead of the salsa.

❊ Replace the sea bass with salmon or cod.

>> MIX IT UP:

>> MIX IT UP:

* Prawns/shrimp or salmon would work well instead of white fish. Go all out like they do in some parts of Mexico and use lobster tail too!
* Pulled jackfruit would work really well as a vegan option.
* Leave out the tortillas and use the lettuce leaves as a wrap.

Fish Tacos with Charred Corn and Spring Onions, Chunky Guacamole and Crispy Lettuce

A bright, fresh and healthy second-trimester-friendly dish. This recipe is my take on the traditional Mexican fish tacos, although here I'm using the more readily available haddock instead of red snapper. Rubbing the corn with spices and lime is a total game-changer — especially if, like me, you were brought up on just butter!

SERVES 2–3
Prep time 15 minutes
Cook time: 10 minutes

* FAMILY FRIENDLY

Ingredients

Juice of 2 limes

1 teaspoon dried oregano

1 teaspoon ground cumin

1 teaspoon ground coriander

1 teaspoon paprika

1 teaspoon cayenne pepper

2 haddock fillets, about 200g/7oz each (or any firm white fish, such as cod, hake or basa)

A knob of butter

2 corn on the cob

A bunch of spring onions/scallions, outer skin removed

2 avocados, peeled, destoned and diced

½ large vine tomato, diced

1 red chilli, deseeded and diced

A bunch of coriander/cilantro, leaves chopped

12 iceberg lettuce leaves (or romaine or something similar)

8–9 whole-wheat tortillas

Salt

1 Preheat the oven to 180°C/350°F/Gas 4.

2 Squeeze the juice of 1½ limes into a bowl and add the oregano, cumin, ground coriander, paprika and cayenne pepper and mix well. Place the haddock fillets on a baking sheet and coat with half of the spice mixture. Sprinkle with a pinch of salt and bake for 10 minutes.

3 Meanwhile, melt the butter in a frying pan over a high heat. Add the corn on the cob, pour over the rest of the spice mixture and cook for 10 minutes, turning frequently. Halfway through cooking add the spring onions/scallions.

4 Next, make the guacamole. In a bowl, mix the avocados with the juice of the remaining lime half. Add the tomato, chilli and some chopped coriander/cilantro leaves. Roughly mash.

5 Remove the fish from the oven, flake into large chunks and sprinkle with some chopped coriander. Serve alongside the lettuce leaves, tortillas, corn on the cobs, spring onions and the rest of the coriander.

Thyme-infused Polenta with Shiitake Mushrooms, Courgette and a Garlic Sauce

Polenta is a good option if you're looking for a change from lentils, pasta or rice. This creamy polenta goes so well with the texture of the shiitake mushrooms and courgettes/zucchini all mixed together with the delicious garlicky sauce. Super quick and easy to make, this is a great plant-based midweek dinner for the second trimester.

SERVES 2
Prep time: 10 minutes
Cook time: 15 minutes

✳ VEGAN/VEGETARIAN
✳ FAMILY FRIENDLY, just use baby-friendly stock

Ingredients

200g/7oz/¾ cup quick-cook polenta/cornmeal
450ml/15fl oz/2 cups hot vegetable stock
8–10 thyme sprigs, leaves chopped
A knob of butter (or a plant-based alternative)
2 shallots, diced
2 garlic cloves, finely chopped
2 courgettes/zucchini, cut into bite-size pieces
200g/7oz shiitake mushrooms

>> **MIX IT UP:**
✳ Aubergine/eggplant would work well here too.
✳ Add some chicken strips for a meat option.
✳ Replace the polenta/cornmeal with risotto rice or pearl barley.

1 Place the polenta/cornmeal into a saucepan. Reserving 50ml of the stock, pour the rest into the pan and stir well. Cook for 5 minutes, stirring well to ensure no lumps form, until the texture becomes paste-like. Add almost all of the thyme (reserve 1–2 sprigs) and mix into the polenta. Set aside and keep warm.

2 Melt the butter in a pan over a high heat. Add the shallots and cook for 2 or 3 minutes before adding in the garlic. Cook for another 30 seconds then add the courgettes and shiitake mushrooms and cook for a further 3–4 minutes.

3 Remove the shiitake mushrooms and courgettes from the pan and set aside so that just the garlic and shallots remain in the pan. Add the remaining stock to the pan and cook on a high heat for 1–2 minutes so the liquid reduces before taking the pan off the heat.

4 Spread the polenta out on a plate. Top with the shitake mushrooms and courgettes. Spoon over the sauce from the pan and top with the leaves from the remaining thyme.

Roasted Asparagus and Peppers with Sweet Potato Fries, Feta and a Spicy Tahini Dressing

Tahini isn't just for making hummus; it's so versatile — and healthy too. Here I've created a delicious spicy tahini sauce that just screams out for the roasted veg to be dipped in it. Great for a light lunch or sharing meal, it works well with many different veggies.

SERVES 2

Prep time: 15 minutes
Cook time: 30 minutes

✻ VEGETARIAN, and leave out the feta for VEGAN
✻ FAMILY FRIENDLY, just leave out the dressing for baby

Ingredients

3–4 sweet potatoes, cut into thick chip shapes
3 teaspoons olive oil
2–3 red, green or yellow peppers (preferably a mix), cored, deseeded and sliced
12 asparagus spears, woody ends removed and sliced into 2 or 3
1 garlic clove, crushed and grated
3 teaspoons tahini
1 teaspoon white wine vinegar
Juice of 1 lemon
1 teaspoon sriracha or chilli flakes
100g/3½oz/⅔ cup feta cheese, crumbled
A few parsley sprigs, leaves chopped
Salt

1 Preheat the oven to 200°C/400°F/Gas 6.

2 Place the sweet potatoes in a roasting pan, add a teaspoon of the oil and pinch of salt. Toss well. Roast for 30 minutes until golden.

3 Place the peppers and asparagus in a separate roasting pan, add a teaspoon of the oil and a pinch of salt, then toss well. Roast for 20 minutes.

4 Meanwhile, make the spicy tahini dressing. In a bowl, mix together the garlic, tahini, vinegar, remaining olive oil and lemon juice. Add the sriracha and a pinch of salt. Mix well, using a few drops of water to loosen, if required.

5 Remove the vegetables and sweet potato fries from the oven and mix in a bowl. Scatter over the feta, then drizzle with the dressing. Sprinkle with the parsley and serve.

>> **MIX IT UP:**
✻ Swap the feta for some cooked halloumi or paneer, or replace with tofu.
✻ Add a runny egg on top for extra protein.
✻ Roasted courgettes/zucchini, artichokes, carrots, spring onions/scallions and aubergine/eggplant would also work well.

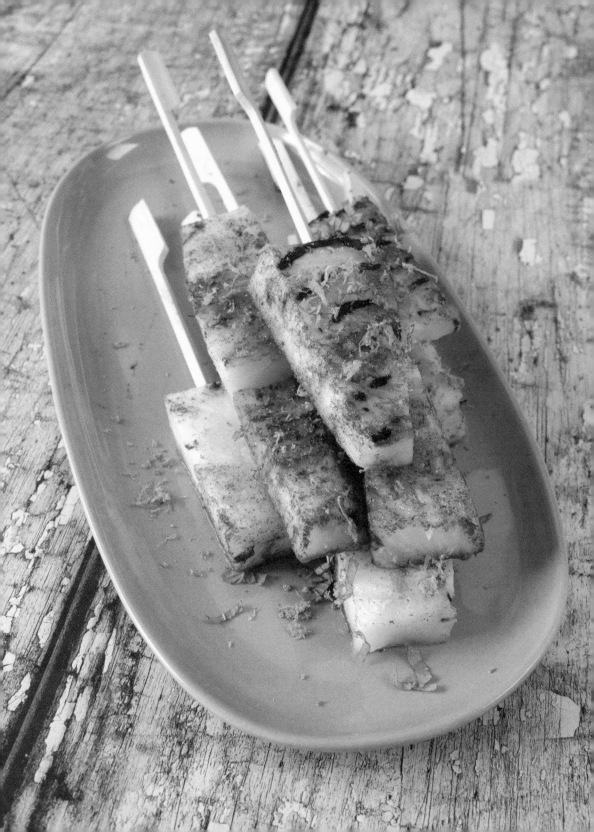

Brazilian Grilled Pineapple with Maple Syrup and Cinnamon

My absolute favourite way to eat pineapple is to do as the Brazilians do and grill it. These are so easy and fun to make and great to enjoy on a hot day. I love the combination of sweet maple syrup and pineapple, tangy lime and fresh mint, this is probably my favourite sweet dish in the book. This recipe works best with a dozen or so wooden skewers, but no biggie if you don't have any.

SERVES 4
Prep time: 10 minutes
Cook time: 20 minutes

✳ FAMILY FRIENDLY, but no maple syrup for under-1s

Ingredients

1 pineapple, outer skin removed and chopped into rectangles measuring roughly 3cm x 10cm/1in x 4in
2 tablespoons maple syrup
2 teaspoons cinnamon
A handful fresh mint leaves, chopped
Zest of 1 lime

1 Skewer the pineapple rectangles. Mix together in a bowl the cinnamon and maple syrup.

2 Pour the mixture over the pineapple pieces ensuring all sides are covered.

3 Cook in a grill pan for 3–4 minutes per wide side then remove from the heat.

4 Place on a plate, then top with the mint and lime zest.

>> **MIX IT UP:**
✳ These would make the perfect accompaniment to a few scoops of ice cream or yogurt.
✳ Swap the pineapple for halved bananas.
✳ Add some raisins or crushed nuts to the pan while grilling the pineapples for extra texture.

Lemon and Basil-Infused Yogurt, Figs, Fresh Berries, Almonds and Honey

I made this dish a lot in Anni's second trimesters. Mixing lemon zest and basil into yogurt takes it to a whole new level as it's deliciously tangy and such a great base for the fruit and almonds, all rounded off with some honey. A lovely little treat that contains protein, fibre and lots of vitamins for mum-to-be and baby.

SERVES 1–2
Prep time: 10 minutes

✱ FAMILY FRIENDLY, but no honey for under-1s

Ingredients
200g/7oz/scant 1 cup Greek yogurt (or a plant-based alternative)
Zest of 1 lemon
Small handful of basil leaves, torn
2–3 figs, halved
100g/3½oz fresh berries (such as strawberries, raspberries and/or blueberries)
2 tablespoons chopped almonds
2 tablespoons honey

1 Spoon the yogurt into a wide bowl. Reserving a pinch of the lemon zest, mix the rest with the yogurt and half the basil.

2 Place the figs and berries on top of the yogurt. Sprinkle over the chopped almonds, reserved lemon zest and remaining basil.

3 Drizzle with the honey and serve.

> > **MIX IT UP:**
> ✱ So many possibilities! Any fruit works well here, especially apples and pears.
> ✱ Try adding some granola or fresh oats.
> ✱ Stir in some dried raisins and cranberries too.

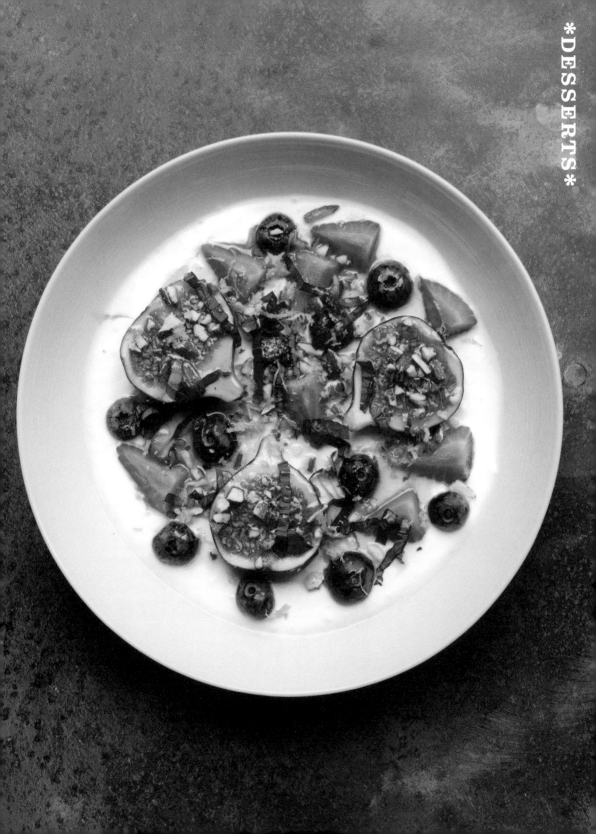

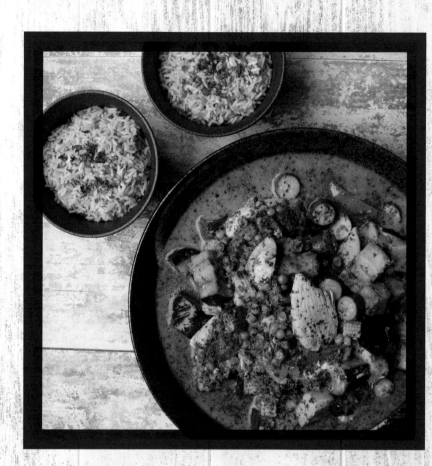

CHAPTER 3:
The Get-Your-Game-Face-On Trimester
(weeks 27 – 40+)

Eating Well in the Get-Your-Game-Face-On Trimester

And just like that, the carefree days of eating the rainbow in the honeymoon trimester fade into the distance, to be replaced by endless to-do lists, shopping for clothes and furniture, birth classes and the feeling that this is all getting very real. Well, for us it did anyway, and the beginning of the third trimester was a bit of a wakeup call for both of us to start getting ready for our new addition!

Baby is beginning to grow quite a bit by this point, which means mum-to-be is also beginning to grow quite a bit. To support that growth, protein- and iron-rich foods continue to be important in terms of generating red blood cells and supporting brain development as well as providing energy for mum-to-be. Again, it's important to say that as long as mum-to-be is taking her recommended vitamin supplements, there is nothing specific that absolutely has to be eaten during this stage but as the body puts the finishing touches to its masterpiece, foods rich in vitamins A and C and calcium become more important. They support bone and teeth development as well as contribute towards healthy gums, skin and good vision.

Baby's growth means that in most cases mum-to-be should be eating an extra 200 calories a day in the third trimester. See the next page for some ideas on what this may look like. However, baby's growth means there's less room inside mum-to-be and her appetite can be affected. She may want to eat less at each meal but more regularly, so one idea could be to have slightly smaller versions of three meals a day and then supplement that with mid-morning and afternoon snacks.

It's worth pointing out that up until this point, we partners have had quite an easy ride. As birth draws nearer, it's a good idea for those involved with the pregnancy and birth to eat well too and start making sure that we are also eating energy-rich foods as we're going to need it!

What does an extra 200 calories look like?

The whole "eating for two" myth is total rubbish. If mum-to-be is enjoying an active pregnancy, then in the third trimester (and only in the third trimester) she should look to eat an extra 200 calories a day to support baby's growth. This could be an avocado, an apple and a handful of nuts, a portion of wholegrain cereal with milk and raisins, or a boiled egg on toast — so it really isn't that much at all.

Getting ready

The third trimester is a great time to start batch-cooking and stocking the freezer with healthy, energy-rich foods to eat in the first few weeks of baby being home. See the spotlight section of this chapter for more tips but in general, as you start thinking about getting the hospital bag ready, start stocking the freezer too. Good luck!

What to focus on

>> **VITAMIN A:** carrots, sweet potatoes, milk and cheese, eggs, oily fish and yogurt.

>> **VITAMIN C:** citrus fruits, sweet potatoes, broccoli, cauliflower, strawberries, peppers, chillies and kale.

>> **CALCIUM:** milk, cheese and other dairy, leafy green vegetables like spinach, kale, cabbage, etc, beans and lentils, almonds, sesame seeds and edamame.

SPOTLIGHT:

Focus on Batch-Cooking

Why is batch-cooking so important?

Batch-cooking for the first few months of baby's life isn't just about eating well or saving money on takeaways, it's about time. Quite simply with a new baby to look after (and play with!) as well as all of life's other demands, no one wants to be stuck in the kitchen each evening cooking. There are more important things to do!

When my first child was born I sadly could only take two weeks off work before returning to a full-time job and over an hour of commuting each way (this was pre-covid). When we were both home with baby and I was on paternity leave, it was a magical period where time seemed not to matter. Baby and new Mum slept, and I found lots of time to make good food for us. Returning to work was a big shock for both of us and this was when batch-cooking became essential. The exhausted new parent version of myself was forever thankful to the third trimester me that took the time when he could to batch-cook and fill the freezer.

Pre-baby, batch-cooking is pretty easy. All you do in the weeks leading up to birth is make twice as much as you usually would for dinner then throw the extra in the freezer. Batch-cooking post-baby becomes that much more difficult as you have so many other things to do – so do it now while you can! When baby is here you can then look forward to a hearty, hot, energy-rich meal ready in minutes at a time when new parents could really do with some good home cooking.

Equipment

You can never have too many air-tight containers in my opinion! Stock up and, as well as the usual standard two-portion rectangular boxes, invest in some bigger ones for larger dishes and smaller ones for random sauces, bites, bars, soups and so on. Ice-cube trays are useful for individual sauces and pestos (and you'll need them for weaning anyway). Buy a few larger silicon ice-cube trays (usually used for making whisky ice cubes) as they are that much larger and are a great way of storing slightly bigger sauce and pesto portions. (Again, great for weaning later too.)

Best foods to batch-cook

So many different foods lend themselves to batch-cooking, as do many recipes in this book (as indicated at the start of each relevant recipe). As well as meals such as large traybakes, pasta dishes, casseroles and stews, other dishes like stir-fries, soups, risottos, biryanis and tagines are also great for the freezer. For super-quick meals, you can't beat an ice cube-tray full of homemade pesto ready to stir into pasta – and one tray can give you many portions. With all of the above taken into account, with minimal effort it can be relatively straightforward for a month's worth of midweek dinners to find their way into your freezer.

Defrosting

If you can, I always think it's best to let meals defrost in the fridge before reheating them in the microwave or oven, or on the hob/stove. If you don't want to freeze rice or pasta, you can always cook it fresh while warming up the rest of the dish. Frozen soups can be warmed up in a saucepan over a low heat. Pesto ice cubes can be added as they are; if using for pasta, simply chuck them in the same pan you used to cook the pasta and cook for 2 minutes with a splash of water while the pasta drains. Reheated risotto tastes better when allowed to defrost and then reheated in a pan with a little water, milk or stock.

Poached Eggs, Cavolo Nero and Bacon Muffins

This is designed to be eaten messily with your fingers! Vitamin- and mineral-rich cavolo nero, salty bacon, creamy Parmesan and runny eggs ... A truly decadent dish to spoil mum-to-be with.

SERVES 2
Prep time: 10 minutes
Cook time: 15 minutes

Ingredients
8 long cavolo nero/black kale leaves
a knob of butter (or a plant-based
    alternative)
8 smoked back bacon rashers/slices
1 teaspoon white wine vinegar
    (for cooking the poached eggs)
Salt
4 eggs
2 English muffins
2 tablespoons grated Parmesan cheese
A few chives, chopped, to garnish

1 Cut the tough stem out of the middle of the cavolo nero/black kale so you're left with two long strips. Melt the butter in a pan, add the cavolo nero and cook for about a minute each side. Remove and set aside.

2 Cook the bacon to your preference in the same pan, then keep warm. Don't make it too crispy, though, as you'll need to roll it up shortly!

3 Meanwhile, make your poached eggs. Fill a deep pan with boiling water and add a pinch of salt and the vinegar. Stir the water gently to create movement, which will help the egg white wrap around the yolk. Crack the eggs into the pan and cook for 3–4 minutes before removing with a slotted spoon. I usually poach 2 eggs at a time.

4 Cut the muffins in half and toast them. Place 1–2 cavolo nero leaves inside each bacon rasher and roll up. Place the rolled bacon on the base of the muffins and top with the poached eggs. Sprinkle with grated Parmesan and garnish with the chives.

>> **MIX IT UP:**
✳ Use curly kale or spinach, if you prefer.
✳ Wrap the cavolo nero in grilled courgettes/zucchini instead of bacon.

Fried Eggs over Samphire, Mushrooms and Cherry Tomatoes

Samphire is absolutely packed full of nutrients and tastes delicious. It's so underrated in my opinion! Most fishmongers will have a huge bag of the stuff to sell you on the cheap and while it does go fantastically well with scallops, white fish and so on, it's also lovely with some runny eggs, as here.

SERVES 2
Prep time: 5 minutes
Cook time: 10 minutes

✳ VEGETARIAN
✳ FAMILY-FRIENDLY

Ingredients
150–200g/5½oz–7oz samphire
A knob of butter (or a plant-based
    alternative)
2 shallots, diced
2 garlic cloves, finely chopped
3–4 chestnut/cremini mushrooms,
    sliced
8 cherry tomatoes, quartered
A squeeze of lemon juice
2–4 eggs

1 Place the samphire in a bowl, cover with boiling water for 1 minutes, then drain. This will help remove a lot of the salt from the samphire.

2 Melt the butter in a frying pan over a medium heat, add the shallots and cook for 3 minutes. Add the garlic, mushrooms, samphire and cherry tomatoes and squeeze a little lemon juice into the pan. Cook for a further 5 minutes.

3 Meanwhile, in a separate pan, fry the eggs to your preference.

4 Divide the samphire mixture between 2 plates and top with 1–2 fried eggs per person.

> > **MIX IT UP:**
✳ Add some chilli to the shallots for extra spice.
✳ Grate a bit of cheese over the eggs for extra calcium.
✳ Stir through some green peas for extra vitamins.
✳ Serve on crusty multigrain bread.

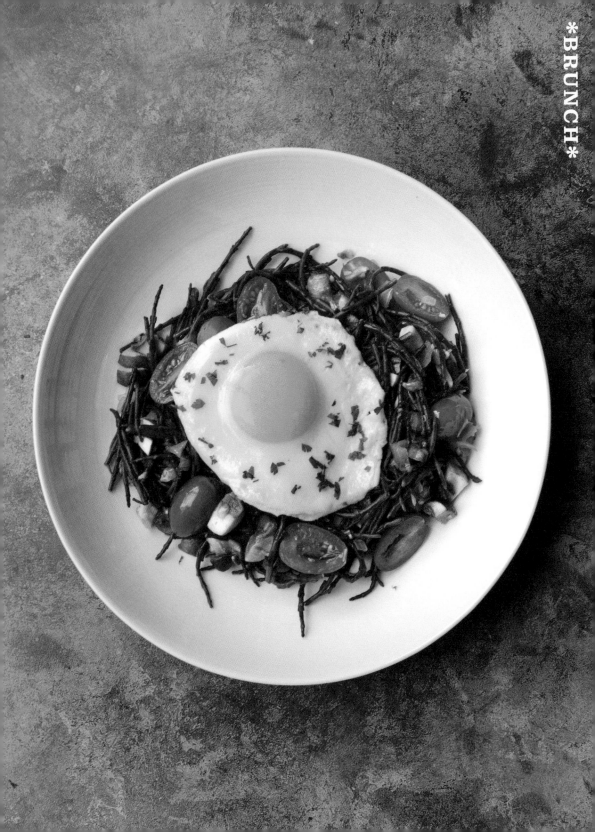

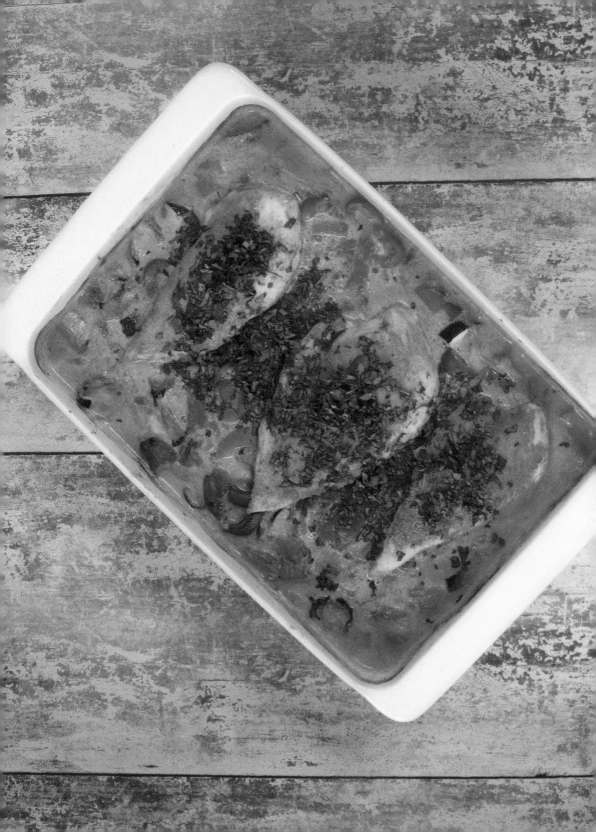

Spiced Chicken and Coconut Traybake

A bright, colourful dish that requires minimal prep, so it's perfect for the third trimester when you've got lots of other things to do! It contains lots of protein for mum-to-be and is high in nutrients from the spices and vegetables. Chuck it all in a dish and whack it in the oven – that's it. This is probably my most-made dish on Instagram.

SERVES 2–3
Prep time: 5 minutes
Cook time: 25 minutes

✳ BATCH-COOK ME!
✳ FAMILY-FRIENDLY,
   just leave out the salt

Ingredients
2 chicken breasts
Juice of 1 lime
1 teaspoon ground cumin
1 teaspoon ground coriander
1 teaspoon ground turmeric
1 onion, diced
2 courgettes/zucchini, diced
1 red pepper, cored, deseeded
   and diced
1 green pepper, cored, deseeded
   and diced
1 x 400g/14oz can of chopped
   tomatoes
1 x 400ml/14fl oz can of coconut milk
250g/9oz/1¼ cups brown basmati
   rice (optional)
A few coriander/cilantro sprigs, leaves
   chopped
Salt

1 Preheat the oven to 180°C/350°F/Gas 4.

2 Slice the chicken breasts in half widthways. Mix together the lime juice, cumin, ground coriander, turmeric and a pinch of salt and rub into each chicken breast. Set aside.

3 Place the onion, courgettes/zucchini and peppers in a deep ovenproof dish. Stir in the canned tomatoes and coconut milk and mix well. Place the chicken breasts on top and bake for 25 minutes.

4 Meanwhile, cook the rice as per the packet instructions, if using.

5 Remove the traybake from the oven and garnish with the chopped coriander/cilantro. Serve with the rice.

>> **MIX IT UP:**
✳ Add in some diced aubergine/eggplant or carrots or top with some grilled beef or cauliflower.
✳ Marinade some firm tofu in the same spice mix and bake separately for 20 minutes before stirring in, or try replacing the chicken with minced/ground pork.

Roasted Cod with Lentils, Cherry Tomatoes and Parsley Oil

This dish is just so simple to make. It makes a great third-trimester recipe as it's packed full of the good stuff. This is on the table in the time it takes to cook the cod, so is a brilliant midweek meal.

SERVES 2
Prep time: 10 minutes
Cook time: 20 minutes

✱ FAMILY-FRIENDLY,
just leave out the salt and use baby-friendly stock

Ingredients

1 lemon
2 cod fillets, around 120g/4¼oz each
5 tablespoons olive oil
1 onion, diced
12 cherry tomatoes, halved
2 garlic cloves, finely chopped
2 x 400g/14oz can of green lentils, drained
75ml/2½fl oz/scant ½ cup vegetable stock
A few parsley sprigs, leaves chopped
Salt and pepper

1 Preheat the oven to 180°C/350°F/Gas 4.

2 Cut half the lemon into thin slices and place on a baking sheet, then place the cod on top. Season the cod and squeeze the remaining lemon half over the fish. Roast for 10–12 minutes until the cod is firm and flakes easily.

3 Meanwhile, heat a tablespoon of the oil in a pan over a low heat. Add the onion and cook for 3 minutes. Add the tomatoes and garlic along with the lentils. Cook for a minute or so before adding in the stock. Cook for a further 3–4 minutes but not for too long, as you want to keep some liquid in the mixture.

4 Stir together the parsley, 4 tablespoons of the oil and a pinch of salt.

5 Divide the lentil mixture into 2 bowls, top with the cod and drizzle over the parsley oil.

>> **MIX IT UP:**
✱ Hake or monkfish would work here instead of the cod.
✱ If you want to replace the fish with a vegetarian option, a few roasted portobello mushrooms would go well with the parsley oil.
✱ Some diced chorizo added to the lentils would be tasty.

Chicken with Creamy Tarragon Mushrooms, Cauliflower Purée and Charred Green Cabbage

Tarragon and chicken are a match made in heaven, as are garlic and mushrooms! I've swapped out potato mash for cauliflower purée to ramp up the nutrients for mum-to-be. A great way of cooking greens is to char them; it creates a delicious smoky taste.

SERVES 2
Prep time: 15 minutes
Cook time: 30 minutes

* FAMILY-FRIENDLY, just leave out the salt and use baby-friendly stock

Ingredients

3 tablespoons olive oil
1 shallot, diced
2 garlic cloves, finely chopped
2 chicken breasts, skin on
200ml/7fl oz/scant 1 cup chicken stock
A bunch of tarragon, chopped
1 head of cauliflower, cut into florets
A knob of butter (or plant-based alternative)
1 tablespoon full-fat/whole milk (or plant-based alternative)
1 green cabbage, outer leaves removed, cut into quarters
100g/3½oz/1½ cups chestnut/cremini mushrooms, sliced
3 tablespoons double/heavy cream (or plant-based alternative)
Salt and pepper

1 Heat a tablespoon of the oil in a frying pan over a medium heat. Add the shallot and cook for a few minutes. Add half the garlic, season the chicken breasts and fry, skin-side down, for 10 minutes. Turn the chicken over, add the stock and some chopped tarragon and cook for a further 15 minutes until cooked through.

2 Meanwhile, cook the cauliflower in a pan of boiling water for 5 minutes. Drain then transfer to a blender with the butter and milk and some of the tarragon. Blitz into a purée.

3 Heat another tablespoon of the oil in a griddle/grill pan over a high heat. Add the cabbage, season and cook for 5 minutes on each side until lightly charred. Remove from the pan and set aside.

4 Heat the remaining tablespoon of oil in the pan over a medium heat. Add the mushrooms and the rest of the garlic and cook for a minute or so, then add the cream and the remaining tarragon. Cook for a few more minutes.

5 Spoon the cauliflower purée onto 2 plates. Slice each chicken breast into 3 pieces and place on the purée, along with any juices from the pan. Spoon the creamy mushrooms over the top. Serve the charred cabbage on the side.

>> **MIX IT UP:**
* Firm white fish, such as cod and haddock,
work well in this dish, but I personally
prefer how the spices go with a meatier fish
like the salmon.
* You could add a few extra vegetables, such
as peas or aubergine/eggplant, to the dish.

Goan Fish Pie

While I do love a traditional fish pie, it is quite heavy and creamy and therefore maybe not a great third-trimester dish when mum-to-be may have less of an appetite. Instead, try this Goan fish pie which features lots of aromatic spices, both to cook the fish in and to mix through the mashed potato. I'm using salmon and prawns/shrimp as they're great for the third trimester, but any fish will do. Make loads for the freezer!

SERVES 2, plus lots for the freezer
Prep time: 20 minutes
Cook time: 40 minutes

* BATCH-COOK ME!
* FAMILY-FRIENDLY

Ingredients

800g/1lb 12oz white potatoes, sliced
1 teaspoon olive oil
1 onion, diced
1 garlic clove, finely chopped
5cm/2in piece of fresh root ginger, peeled and finely chopped
2 teaspoons ground cumin
2 teaspoons ground turmeric
2 teaspoons ground coriander
2 teaspoons garam masala
2 teaspoons mustard seeds
Juice of 1 lime
1 x 400ml/14fl oz can of coconut milk
3–4 salmon fillets, about 150g/5½oz each, cut into bite-sized chunks
A handful of cherry tomatoes, halved
2 large handfuls of spinach leaves, chopped
200g/7oz king prawns/jumbo shrimp
30g/1oz butter (or a plant-based alternative)
A bunch of coriander/cilantro, leaves chopped

1 Heat the oven to 180°C/350°F/Gas 4.

2 Cook the potatoes in a pan of lightly salted boiling water for 10 minutes. Drain and set aside.

3 Meanwhile, heat the oil in a frying pan over a medium heat. Add the onion and cook for 3 minutes. Add the garlic and ginger, then add 1 teaspoon each of the cumin, turmeric, ground coriander, garam masala and mustard seeds and mix well. Add the lime juice and a third of the coconut milk and stir.

4 Add the salmon to the pan, along with the rest of the coconut milk and cook for 5 minutes.

5 Add the tomatoes along with the spinach. Stir in the prawns/shrimp and cook for 3 minutes until pink. Remove the pan from the heat and transfer the contents into a bowl.

6 Melt the butter in the same pan over a medium heat, add the remaining spices and stir well for a minute or so. Add the potatoes, then mash. Stir in the fresh coriander/cilantro.

7 Spoon the fish mixture into an ovenproof dish and, using a fork, spread out the mash on top. Bake for around 20 minutes until golden.

Veg-Packed Thai Green Curry

I've dialled down the spice and increased the vegetables for this homemade Thai green curry. There's no need to buy a curry paste, as you can make this fresh one in minutes. This dish is a real family favourite and works with chicken, prawns/shrimp, tofu or just loads of veg.

SERVES 2
Prep time: 10 minutes
Cook time: 20 minutes

✳ BATCH-COOK ME!

Ingredients

250g/9oz/1¼ cups brown basmati rice
A bunch of coriander/cilantro
1 green chilli, deseeded and diced
2 lemongrass stalks, chopped
5cm/2in piece of fresh root ginger, peeled
1 shallot
1 teaspoon fish sauce
1 teaspoon brown sugar
Juice of 1 lime
1 x 400ml/14fl oz can of coconut milk
2 chicken breasts, sliced
75g/2½oz/⅓ cup frozen peas
1 aubergine/eggplant, diced
4 baby corn, chopped (or 75g/2½oz/⅓ cup frozen sweetcorn)
4 baby courgettes/zucchini (or 1 large courgette), sliced
1 red pepper, cored, deseeded and diced

1 Cook the rice as per the packet instructions.

2 Meanwhile, place the coriander/cilantro, chilli, lemongrass, ginger, shallot, fish sauce, brown sugar and lime juice in a blender and blitz until it's a chunky paste.

3 Put 2 tablespoons of the paste into a large pan over a medium heat, along with a third of the coconut milk. Stir well. Add the chicken and cook for 5 minutes.

4 Add the remaining paste and coconut milk to the pan, along with the vegetables. Cook for a further 8–10 minutes before serving alongside the rice.

>> **MIX IT UP:**
✳ Swap in prawns/shrimp or tofu for the chicken. Add some mushrooms and cherry tomatoes for extra vitamins, or an extra chilli to the paste for more heat.
✳ If you make a larger batch of the paste, you can freeze it or it will keep in the fridge for 3–4 days.

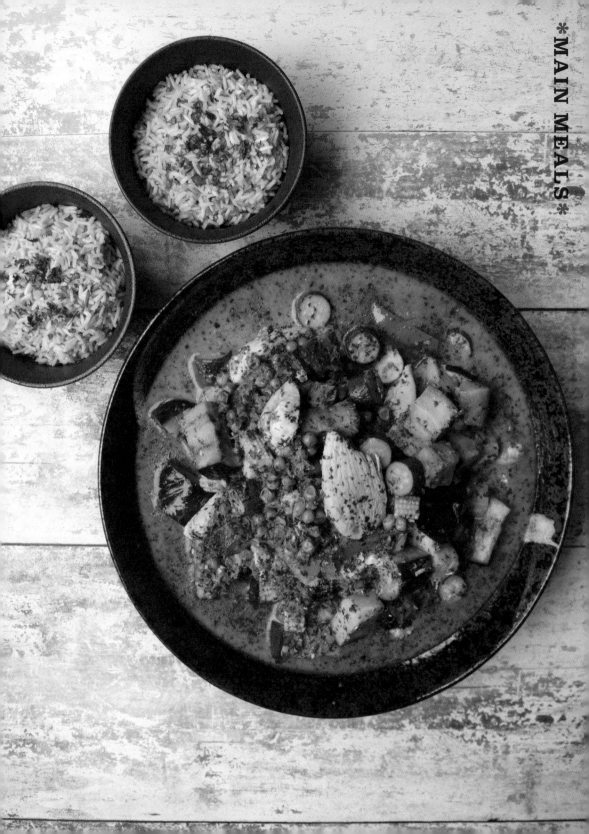

Lamb, Apricot and Pomegranate Tagine

This takes a little while but is worth it: melt-in-the-mouth lamb and sweet fruits, finished with pomegranate. Make this on one of those long days of waiting for baby. It's also perfect for freezing.

SERVES 2, plus some for the freezer
Prep time: 15 minutes
Cook time: 70 minutes

✳ BATCH-COOK ME!
✳ FAMILY-FRIENDLY,
  just leave out the salt and use
  baby-friendly stock

Ingredients

1 tablespoon olive oil
400g/14oz lamb neck, cut into
  2½cm/1in cubes
1 onion, chopped
1 teaspoon paprika
1 teaspoon ground cumin
1 teaspoon ground cinnamon
3 garlic cloves, finely chopped
1 tablespoon honey
2 carrots, diced
1 aubergine/eggplant, cut into
  2.5cm/1in cubes
1 x 400g/14oz can chopped tomatoes
1 x 400g/14oz can of chickpeas/
  garbanzo beans, drained
200g/7oz/1⅔ cups dried apricots
50g/1¾oz/⅓ cup raisins
500ml/17fl oz/2 cups lamb stock
200g/7oz/1⅓ cups couscous
Seeds from ½ pomegranate
Small handful of coriander/cilantro
  leaves, chopped
Salt

1 First, brown the lamb. Heat the oil in a heavy-based casserole dish over a high heat. Season the lamb with salt and add to the dish. Cook for a few minutes until nicely browned. Remove and set aside.

2 Add the onion to the same dish along with the paprika, cumin and cinnamon. Stir well to ensure the onion is covered in the spices, then add the garlic and honey.

3 Add the carrot and aubergine/eggplant along with the canned tomatoes, chickpeas/garbanzo beans, apricots and raisins. Stir the lamb back in and pour over the stock. Cover and cook for about an hour until the lamb is tender, topping up with stock or boiling water if needed.

4 When the lamb is nearly cooked, make the couscous as per the packet instructions.

5 Remove the dish from the heat and top with the pomegranate seeds and coriander. Serve with the couscous alongside.

>> **MIX IT UP:**
✳ For a vegan option, replace the lamb with more aubergine, or red peppers, butter/lima beans or black-eyed beans/peas.
✳ Increase the heat by adding a little chilli powder or cayenne pepper.
✳ Serve with yogurt and flatbreads, rice or quinoa instead of the couscous.

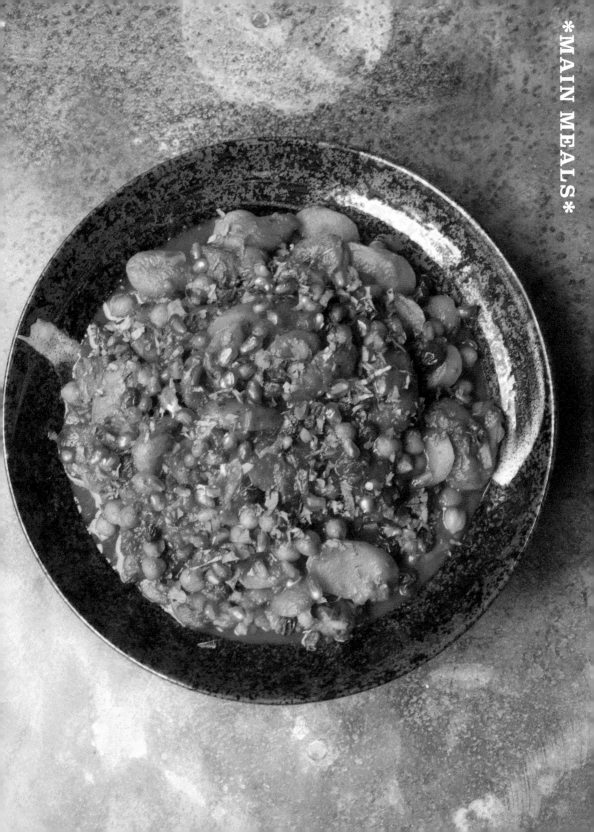

Creamy Coconut Dhal with Sweet Potato and Indian-spiced Monkfish Tails

This creamy dhal with a hint of spice makes a great date-night meal if you're looking for something a bit special towards the end of mum-to-be's pregnancy. It's also a really healthy dish with the combination of the lentils, sweet potatoes and meaty monkfish tails — all great pregnancy superfoods. The dhal is perfect for batch-cooking too.

SERVES 2

Prep time: 10 minutes

Cook time: 20 minutes

✱ BATCH-COOK ME!

✱ FAMILY-FRIENDLY,
   just leave out the salt

Ingredients

2 teaspoons olive oil

1 shallot, diced

1 garlic clove, crushed

2 teaspoons ground turmeric

2 teaspoons ground coriander

2 teaspoons ground cumin

2 teaspoons mustard seeds

2 x 400g/14oz cans of green lentils, drained

1 x 400ml/14fl oz can of coconut milk

2–3 sweet potatoes, diced

2 large tomatoes, chopped

A few coriander/cilantro sprigs, leaves chopped

2 monkfish tails

Juice of 1 lemon

A knob of butter (or a plant-based alternative)

Salt

1 Heat a teaspoon of the oil in a pan over a medium heat. Add the shallot along with a pinch of salt and cook for 3 minutes. Add the garlic along with a teaspoon each of the turmeric, ground coriander, cumin and mustard seeds. Cook for a further minute.

2 Add the lentils to the pan, then mix in the coconut milk. Add the sweet potato and tomatoes and cook for 20 minutes. Towards the end of cooking, stir in the fresh coriander/cilantro.

3 Meanwhile, mix the remaining spices together, then rub into the monkfish tails. Squeeze over the lemon juice. Heat the remaining teaspoon of the oil in a separate pan and cook the monkfish for 6–7 minutes. Turn the fish over, add the butter and cook for a further 3 minutes. Remove from the heat and leave to rest for 2–3 minutes.

4 Spoon the dhal into a shallow bowl, then cut each monkfish tail in half and place on top, drizzling any juices from the pan over the fish before serving.

>> **MIX IT UP:**
* Swap the monkfish for either cod,
haddock or seabass (roast the cod or
haddock for 10 minutes in the oven, but
pan-fry the seabass for 4–5 minutes).
* For a vegan option, rub the marinade into
a cauliflower steak and roast in the oven
for 20 minutes.

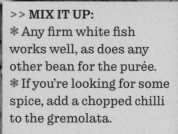

>> **MIX IT UP:**
* Any firm white fish
works well, as does any
other bean for the purée.
* If you're looking for some
spice, add a chopped chilli
to the gremolata.

Cod with Pea and Cannellini Bean Purée and Gremolata

This is a bit of a play on battered fish and mushy peas. The gremolata adds some texture and a refreshing blast of lemon, while the pea and bean purée is a great substitute for mash and is full of nutrients. This is another quick dish to make and one I made a lot for my wife in her third trimesters. The gremolata lasts for a few days in the refrigerator and is great for adding to soups and salads too.

SERVES 2
Prep time: 10 minutes
Cook time: 15 minutes

* FAMILY-FRIENDLY,
   just leave out the salt and use
   baby-friendly stock

Ingredients

1 lemon

2 cod fillets, about 150g/5½oz each

2 teaspoons of olive oil

1 onion, diced

50ml/2fl oz/3–4 tablespoons
   vegetable stock

200g/7oz/1 cup frozen peas

1 x 400g/14oz can of cannellini
   beans, drained

A knob of butter (or a plant-based
   alternative)

1 slice of wholegrain bread, toasted

1 garlic clove

A few parsley sprigs

Salt

1 Preheat the oven to 180°C/350°F/Gas 4.

2 Zest the lemon and set aside. Slice the lemon and place four slices on a baking tray, then place the two pieces of cod on the lemon. Season and bake for 10 minutes.

3 Heat a teaspoon of the oil in a pan over a medium heat. Add the onion, season and fry for a few minutes. Add the stock, peas, cannellini beans and butter and cook for 5 minutes. Blend the contents of the pan until you have a smooth purée.

4 For the gremolata, place the toasted bread, garlic, lemon zest, parsley and remaining oil in a blender and whizz until smooth.

5 Place the purée on 2 plates. Remove the cod from the oven and place them on top of the purée. Spoon over the gremolata.

Smoked Salmon Poke Bowl

For when you can't have sushi! My wife really missed eating sushi during her pregnancy, so I decided to make a poke bowl using smoked salmon instead of raw salmon and it went down really well. As long as the smoked salmon has been previously frozen (most shop-bought smoked salmon has) it's absolutely fine to eat in pregnancy, and when combined with the edamame beans and avocado – two delicious superfoods – it makes a really healthy dish.

SERVES 2
Prep time: 10 minutes
Cook time: 20 minutes

✳ FAMILY-FRIENDLY

Ingredients

200g/7oz/generous 1 cup brown rice
5cm/2in piece of fresh root ginger, peeled and finely grated
1 garlic clove, crushed
2 tablespoons soy sauce
1 teaspoon rice wine vinegar or red wine vinegar
1 teaspoon sesame oil
1 teaspoon honey
50g/1¾oz/⅓ cup fresh or frozen edamame beans
1 avocado, peeled, destoned and diced
Juice of 1 lime
200g/7oz smoked salmon, sliced
1 teaspoon black sesame seeds
1 teaspoon white sesame seeds

1 Cook the rice as per the packet instructions, then drain and set aside to cool.

2 In a bowl, mix the ginger, garlic, soy sauce, vinegar, sesame oil and honey.

3 If using frozen edamame beans, place them in a bowl and cover with hot water. Leave for a few minutes to defrost.

4 Spoon the rice into a bowl. Cover a quarter of the top of the rice with the edamame. Cover another quarter with the diced avocado and squeeze the lime juice over it to stop it browning. Arrange the salmon over another quarter and spoon over as much of the soy sauce mixture as you want. Sprinkle the sesame seeds over the salmon before serving.

> **>> MIX IT UP:**
> ✳ Add a little hot sauce to the soy sauce mixture or some diced chilli to the avocado.
> ✳ Swap the smoked salmon for prawns/shrimp or tofu.
> ✳ Swap the edamame for peas, if you prefer.
> ✳ Add a little nori seaweed to the bowl.

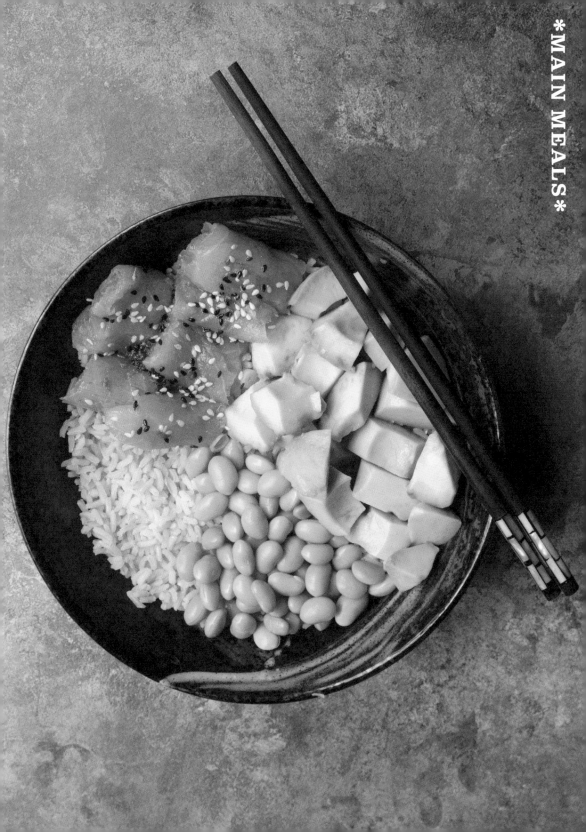

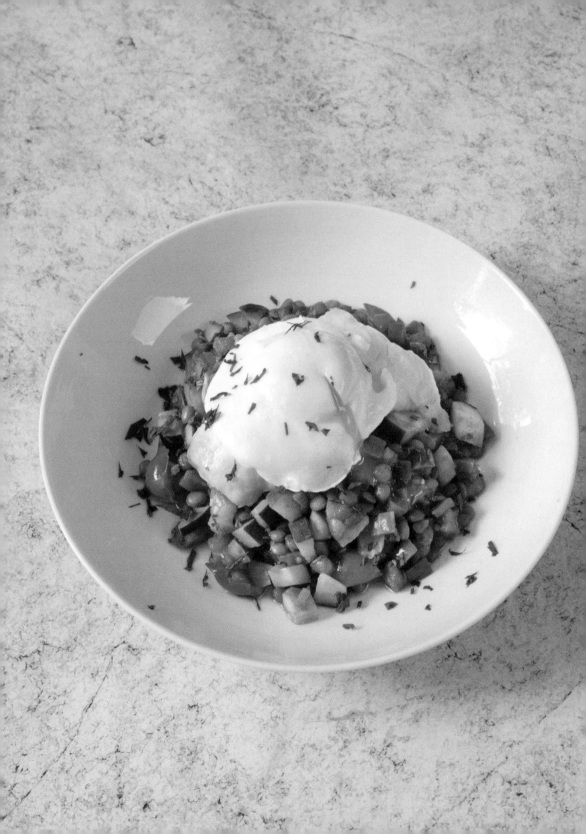

Roasted Haddock, Smoky Lentil and Veg Stew and Poached Eggs

Everything mum-to-be needs is in this dish, and I love how the yolk oozes into the smoky stew! Any white fish works instead of haddock.

SERVES 2

Prep time: 15 minutes

Cook time: 20 minutes

* FAMILY-FRIENDLY,
just leave out the salt

Ingredients

1 teaspoon olive oil

1 shallot, diced

2 garlic cloves, finely chopped

1 teaspoon ground cumin

1 teaspoon smoked paprika

2 peppers, preferably different colours,
cored, deseeded and diced

1 courgette/zucchini, diced

1 x 400g/14oz can chopped tomatoes

1 lemon

2 haddock fillets, about 140g/5oz each

1 x 400g/14oz can green lentils,
drained

2 handfuls of spinach leaves, chopped

2 eggs

1 teaspoon vinegar

A few chives, chopped

Salt

>> **MIX IT UP:**
* For a vegan option, cook
a cauliflower steak in a
teaspoon each of cumin
and paprika mixed with oil.
* Top with crumbled feta
for extra calcium.

1 Preheat the oven to 180°C/350°F/Gas 4.

2 Heat a teaspoon of the oil over a medium heat. Add the shallot and cook for a few minutes. Add the garlic along with a pinch of salt, the cumin and the smoked paprika and cook for a minute. Add the mixed peppers and courgette/zucchini and cook for 5 minutes.

3 Add the tomatoes to the pan and cook for a further 10 minutes.

4 Meanwhile, cut 4 slices from one half of lemon and place on a baking sheet. Arrange the haddock on top, squeeze over the remaining lemon and bake for 10–12 minutes.

5 Add the lentils to the pan along with the spinach and reduce the heat to low.

6 To make the poached eggs, bring a deep, wide pan of water to the boil. Reduce to a simmer, add the vinegar and stir gently. Crack the eggs into the pan (the movement of the stirred water wraps the egg white around the yolk) and cook for 3–4 minutes. Remove with a slotted spoon and place on paper towels.

7 To serve, divide the stew between 2 bowls and place a haddock fillet on top of each portion. Add a poached egg to each bowl and garnish with the chives.

>> **MIX IT UP:**
* If you aren't a fan of cauliflower rice, swap it out for brown rice or noodles.
* Diced chicken or pork would work well with the sauce, as would some baked salmon.
* Add some chopped chilli to the sauce for more of a kick.

Tofu, Kale and Cashew Stir-fry with Roasted Cauliflower Rice

Roasted cauliflower rice really elevates a dish in my opinion. It's a great low-carb option and I love how the smokiness runs through the dish, perfectly complementing the stir-fried vegetables. Cooking the tofu in the oven first means it'll stay firm when you stir-fry it.

SERVES 2
Prep time: 15 minutes
Cook time: 25 minutes

* VEGETARIAN/VEGAN, just use maple syrup instead of honey
* FAMILY-FRIENDLY

Ingredients

200g/7oz/¾ cup firm tofu, cut into 2cm/¾in cubes
1 head of cauliflower, cut into florets
4 tablespoons soy sauce
1 teaspoon rice wine vinegar or white wine vinegar
1 teaspoon honey
1 teaspoon cornflour/cornstarch
5cm/2in piece of fresh root ginger, peeled and grated
2 garlic cloves, crushed
A handful of cashew nuts
1 teaspoon sesame oil
1 shallot, diced
8 chestnut/cremini mushrooms, chopped
1 green pepper, cored, deseeded and diced
A few handfuls of kale, tough stalks removed, roughly chopped
1 spring onion/scallion, sliced
1 teaspoon sesame seeds

1 Preheat the oven to 180°C/350°F/Gas 4.

2 Place the tofu on a baking sheet and bake for 15 minutes.

3 Meanwhile, place the cauliflower in a blender or food processor and blitz for a few seconds until the cauliflower resembles and has a rice/sand-like texture. Spoon into a greased baking pan and roast in the oven for 20 minutes, stirring occasionally.

4 Make the sauce. In a bowl, mix together the soy sauce, vinegar, honey and cornflour/cornstarch. Add the ginger and half of the garlic, stir well, then set aside.

5 In a hot frying pan over a medium heat, dry-fry the cashew nuts for 2–3 minutes, then remove and set aside.

6 Heat a teaspoon of the oil in a pan over a medium heat. Add the shallot and cook for 2 minutes. Add the remaining garlic and the mushrooms and pepper and cook for 5 minutes. Remove the tofu from the oven and add to the pan with the soy sauce mixture and cashew nuts. Cook for 2 minutes before adding the kale and cooking for a further 2 minutes.

7 Spoon the cauliflower rice into bowls. Top with the tofu stir-fry and garnish with the sliced spring onion/scallion and sesame seeds.

Gambas al Ajillo

A super-quick garlicky dish to eat either at the end of a long day or on the go while pacing round the house waiting for baby. Prawns/shrimp are little bites of pure protein, so are a fantastic food for the third trimester when mum-to-be needs to increase her protein intake but might not have a very big appetite.

SERVES 2
Prep time: 5 minutes
Cook time: 5 minutes

Ingredients

2 tablespoons olive oil

4–5 garlic cloves, crushed

1 red chilli, diced (deseeded for less spice), or 1 tablespoon dried chilli/hot pepper flakes

1 teaspoon paprika

300g/10½oz raw peeled prawns/shrimp

Juice of 1 lemon

A few parsley sprigs, leaves chopped

Salt

1 Heat the oil in a pan over a medium heat. Add the garlic, chilli, paprika and a pinch of salt. Cook for 2 minutes.

2 Add the prawns/shrimp to the pan along with another pinch of salt and the lemon juice. Cook for another 2–3 minutes until the prawns turn pink.

3 Sprinkle over the parsley and serve immediately.

> > **MIX IT UP:**
> * The spice is optional, so swap the chilli for a diced shallot or spring onions/scallions if you like.
> * Serve with some crusty buttered bread. Mmmm.

Chocolate-Dipped Strawberries

It's so easy to make chocolate-dipped strawberries — you can do it in under 10 minutes! They're great for a snack and an energy burst when mum-to-be needs it. Make loads and keep them in the fridge for 48 hours … if they last!

SERVES AS MANY AS YOU WANT!

Prep time: 10 minutes, plus 15 minutes chilling time

Ingredients

1 x 200g/1oz bar of good-quality chocolate (white, milk or dark, as you prefer)

1 punnet of strawberries

2–3 tablespoons desiccated coconut

1 Bring a saucepan of water to the boil and place a heatproof bowl over it, making sure the bottom of the bowl doesn't touch the water. Break up the chocolate into the bowl and stir when it begins to melt.

2 When all the chocolate has melted, dip a strawberry into the chocolate. Remove, sprinkle with desiccated coconut and place on parchment paper. Repeat until all the chocolate or strawberries have gone, then refrigerate for at least 15 minutes.

>> **MIX IT UP:**
* Other fruits work really well, including mango, papaya, banana and blueberries.
* Melt some white chocolate in addition to milk or dark and double-dip to create two colours.
* Sprinkle some crushed pistachios or almonds over the fruit instead of the coconut.

Date, Almond, Chocolate and Tahini Energy Balls

The dates, oats and almonds make these balls great for a slow-release energy boost when mum-to-be needs it most in those last remaining weeks. Make a load for the freezer and just take out a few at a time to keep in the refrigerator when needed.

MAKES AROUND 18 BALLS

Prep time: 15 minutes, plus
2 hours chilling time

* BATCH-COOK ME!
* VEGETARIAN
* FAMILY-FRIENDLY, as long as there are no nut allergies

Ingredients

200g/7oz/1⅓ cups destoned
Medjool dates, chopped
3 tablespoons cocoa powder
2 tablespoons smooth peanut butter
50g/1¾oz/½ cup rolled oats
80g/3oz almonds, chopped
3 tablespoons tahini
4–5 tablespoons desiccated coconut,
for rolling

1 Place the dates in a food processor along with the cocoa powder, peanut butter, oats and almonds. Blend until a sticky mixture forms. Add the tahini then blend again.

2 Roll the mixture into golf-ball-sized balls.

3 Roll the balls in the desiccated coconut, then place in an airtight container in the refrigerator for at least 2 hours before eating.

>> **MIX IT UP:**
* Lots of possibilities here. Instead of tahini, use coconut oil or maple syrup and swap the almonds for cashews.
* Add chocolate chips instead of cocoa powder, chuck in some raisins and roll the balls in sesame seeds instead of coconut.

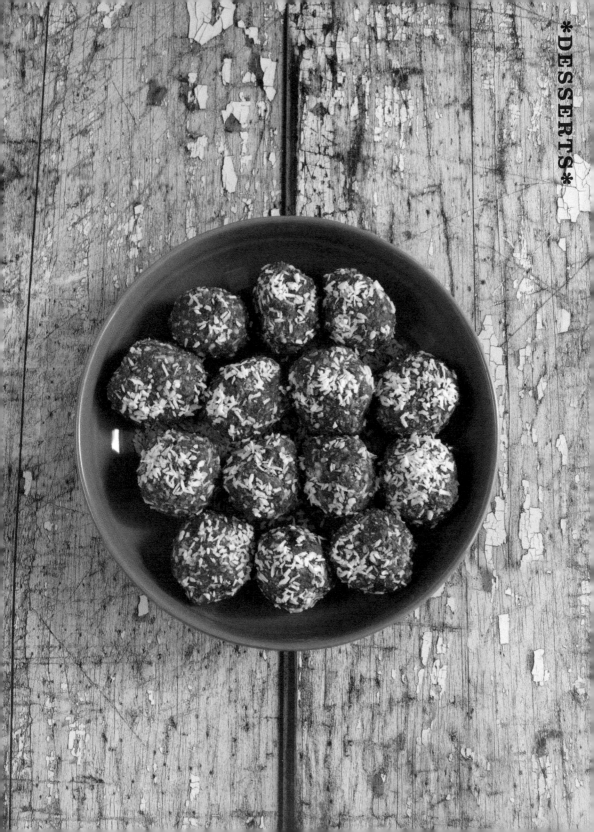

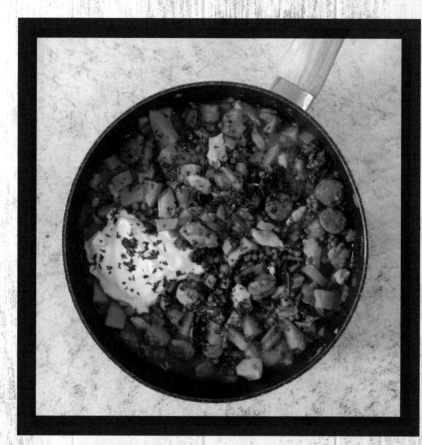

CHAPTER 4:
Feeding Tired
New Parents

Eating Well as a
Tired New Parent

Congratulations! Whether this is your first or fifth, spending time at home with a brand-spanking-new shiny baby is an incredibly special and unforgettable time — not just for Mum but partners and family members too. Whether baby is demanding all your time and energy or you just can't take your eyes off of this tiny human that you made, homemade food understandably isn't a priority right now. Exhaustion means there can be a temptation to resort to shop-bought ready meals and takeaways to keep you going, and while there's nothing wrong with this, they can not only hurt your wallet but may make you feel even more tired and groggy than you do already.*

You're breast- or bottle-feeding every few hours, the washing machine is on a never-ending cycle, baby is only sleeping on you and one of you has probably returned to work, so is unavailable for most of the day. It's fair to say the whole house is feeling pretty tired. This is when any batch-cooking you've done really comes into its own — so if you did any, well done, you! See page 85 for batch-cooking ideas and look out for the batch-cooking highlight on recipes in this chapter and throughout this book.

In general, following a healthy diet and eating lots of energy-rich whole grains, lean protein, pulses and leafy greens, such as those featured in this chapter, will hopefully give you what you need to keep going and approach the 3am feed with a smile! (Maybe.)

---

* Full disclosure: When we brought both our babies home for the first time, we celebrated that night with a take-away pizza and it tasted amazing!

Foods for when new mums are breastfeeding

If Mum has decided to breastfeed, there are certain foods she can eat during this period that not only stimulate milk production but help replace the energy she is burning off. Calcium-rich foods help replace calcium that she passes on in her milk, and iron- and protein-rich foods help give her the energy she needs to get through the day while breastfeeding. A lot of the recipes in this chapter focus on these food groups. For a more detailed breakdown see pages 14, 50 and 84.

One-handed food and snacking

Whether breastfeeding or not, there will be many occasions where one of you will probably find yourself hungry and alone with a sleeping baby on top of you that you'd do anything not to wake.

At these times having some food in the fridge that you can eat with one hand will come in pretty useful. This chapter contains some ideas on how to eat meals alone with one hand and also features numerous recipes for dips, spreads and snacks that one of you can make and leave in the refrigerator for a one-handed snack.

When it comes to nocturnal snacking, there's a great recipe for a chocolate mousse on page 142, and make sure you stock up on hot chocolate!

One-Handed Foods

For most new families, at some point one of the parents will find themselves alone with a small baby for long periods of time. One of you has likely returned to work and any family members that came to help at the beginning have left. During these times it can be hard to make good food for yourself along with all the other things you need to do when home alone with a small baby. Here are a few ideas for some easy-to-eat-with-one-hand dishes that you or your partner can make in advance, so that feeding yourself is something you don't need to worry about. All of these can be made quickly before the working week and left in the fridge for a pick 'n' mix meal.

＊ Pre-make some pesto and boil some pasta for cold pasta salads. Fusilli is the best pasta to eat one-handed and the best to have with pesto because the sauce sticks to the spirals. For pesto recipes see pages 15–18.

＊ Pre-make some 3-minute dips and spreads to either enjoy with cucumber and celery sticks or spread on toast. Top with different nuts and seeds for extra nutrition. For recipes see pages 118–119.

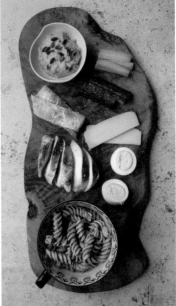

＊ Roast or fry chicken breasts with a squeeze of lemon juice and some chopped rosemary. Either make a batch for the refrigerator (they'll last 48 hours) or freeze after you've cooked them, defrost each morning and eat cold for lunch.

＊ Roast some vegetables such as peppers, courgettes/zucchini and aubergines/eggplant in a few tablespoons of olive oil with some rosemary for 20 minutes. Once cool, refrigerate and eat cold during the week.

＊ Boil a load of eggs at the start of the week and have one a day from the refrigerator.

＊ Pre-chop some vegetables and slice some cheese for a one-handed snack.

Healthy Dips and Spreads for When You Can't Put Baby Down

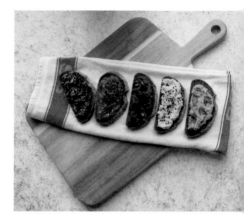

All of these dips are easy to eat with one hand and will keep for 4–5 days in the refrigerator. Eat them as they are with a spoon, spread them on toast, dip with breadsticks or vegetables, put them on top of a jacket potato or stir through soup and pasta. They will keep hunger at bay while baby has a well-deserved snooze on you. And don't worry about dropping any on baby's head, it's all cold and we've all been there!

✳ VEGETARIAN/VEGAN ✳

Beetroot Hummus

A vibrant-coloured hummus made all the better by the addition of the nutrient-rich beetroot/beets.

Ingredients

1 x 400g/14oz can of chickpeas/garbanzo beans, drained ✳ 250g/9oz pre-cooked beetroot/beets, diced ✳ Juice of ½ lemon ✳ A few parsley sprigs, leaves chopped

METHOD

1 Place the chickpeas/garbanzo beans in a food processor. Reserving a tablespoon of the diced beetroot/beets, add the rest to the food processor. Squeeze in the lemon juice and blend until smooth.

2 Top with the reserved beetroot and chopped parsley.

Cannellini, Spinach and Parsley Dip

A really filling dip that tastes especially great in sandwiches.

Ingredients

1 x 400g/14oz can of cannellini beans, drained ✳ Large handful of spinach leaves, chopped ✳ Small handful of parsley leaves ✳ 1 garlic clove ✳ 4 tablespoons olive oil

METHOD

1 Place all of the ingredients in a food processor and blend until smooth. Add a splash or two of water as you go to get your preferred consistency.

Chimichurri

Best known for drizzling over a steak, this spread is delicious on toast for when you want a little heat.

Ingredients
Small handful of parsley ✱ Small handful of coriander/cilantro ✱ 1 green chilli (deseeded, if you prefer) ✱ 1 shallot ✱ 1 garlic clove ✱ 4 tablespoons olive oil ✱ 1 tomato, finely chopped

METHOD

1 Place the parsley and coriander/cilantro (including the stalks) in a food processor. Add the chilli along with the shallot and garlic. Pour in the olive oil.

2 Blend until smooth, adding an additional splash or two of oil as you go to get your preferred consistency. Stir in the tomatoes.

Spanish Tomato and Garlic

Known as *Pan con Tomate* in Spain, the original recipe calls for garlic to be rubbed onto toasted bread, but this isn't the easiest thing to do while holding a baby!

Ingredients
4 ripe tomatoes ✱ 1 garlic clove ✱ A few chives, chopped ✱ Salt

METHOD

1 Place the tomatoes in a food processor along with the garlic and a pinch of salt. Blend until smooth.

2 Sprinkle over the chopped chives.

Miso Hummus

When you've tried salty, earthy miso in your hummus you'll never go back to the original again!

Ingredients
1 x 400g/14oz can of chickpeas/garbanzo beans, drained ✱ 2 tablespoons miso paste ✱ 3 tablespoons sesame oil ✱ Sesame seeds, to garnish

METHOD

1 Place the chickpeas/garbanzo beans in a food processor and add the miso and sesame oil.

2 Blend until smooth, then sprinkle over the sesame seeds.

A Tasty Breakfast Wrap to Eat with One Hand

Eating a cooked breakfast can be tricky if you need to hold a little one at the same time. Equally, if one of you has been up all night with baby, a cooked breakfast is exactly what you need. The answer is to put whatever you want to eat in a wrap and, hey presto, a one-handed hot breakfast to enjoy!

SERVES 1
Prep time: 10 minutes
Cook time: 10 minutes

✳ VEGETARIAN
✳ FAMILY-FRIENDLY

Ingredients
2 teaspoons olive oil ✳ 1 shallot, diced ✳ 1 garlic clove, finely chopped ✳ 1 teaspoon dried oregano ✳ 3–4 chestnut mushrooms, sliced ✳ Handful of spinach leaves, chopped ✳ ½ avocado, peeled, destoned and sliced ✳ 1 whole-wheat tortilla ✳ 2 slices of salami or ham (optional) ✳ 2 eggs, whisked ✳ 2 tablespoons grated Cheddar cheese ✳ Salt

1 Heat a teaspoon of the oil in a pan over a low heat. Add the shallot, season and cook for a few minutes. Add the garlic, along with the oregano and the mushrooms and cook for 2 minutes. Add the spinach and cook for a further minute.

2 Arrange the avocado slices down the centre of the tortilla. Using a slotted spoon, place the contents of the pan on top of the avocado. Add the salami or ham, if using.

3 Pour the whisked eggs into the same pan with the remaining oil and cook until scrambled.

4 Spoon the eggs on top of the salami, sprinkle over the grated Cheddar, wrap it up and devour.

Vegetable Crisps

Get someone to put these in the oven first thing and by mid-morning there'll be enough vegetable crisps to snack on throughout the day. A much better (and tastier) snack then deep-fried potato crisps/chips! There's no need to peel the vegetables but do remove tops and bottoms. These crisps will last for about a day after you've cooked them. These go great with the dips on pages 118–119.

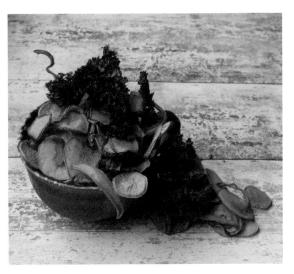

MAKES ENOUGH TO GRAZE ON FOR 1 DAY

Prep time: 15 minutes
Cook time: 75 minutes

✱ VEGAN/VEGETARIAN

Ingredients

1 white potato, very thinly sliced ✱ 1 sweet potato, very thinly sliced ✱ 2–3 raw beetroot/beets, very thinly sliced ✱ 2–3 large carrots, very thinly sliced ✱ A bunch of kale, tough stalks removed, roughly chopped ✱ 1 teaspoon olive oil per vegetable ✱ Salt

1 Preheat the oven to 120°C/250°F/Gas ½ and line 2–3 baking sheets with non-stick baking paper.

2 Place the vegetables in separate bowls, mix each with a teaspoon of olive oil and add a pinch of salt.

3 Spread the potatoes, beetroot/beets and carrots out on the baking sheets, taking care not to overcrowd, so they crisp up nicely, and bake for an hour.

4 Spread the kale out on a baking sheet and bake for 15 minutes to crisp up.

5 Remove from the oven to stop them drying out and eat. Store in an air-tight container for the rest of the day.

Lentil and Vegetable Bolognese

Swapping traditional minced/ground beef for energy-rich lentils is a real game changer, a quick way of cooking Bolognese and one that will leave you feeling less uncomfortably full after eating.

SERVES 2, plus plenty
  for the freezer
Prep time: 10 minutes
Cook time: 30 minutes

✳ BATCH COOK ME!
✳ VEGETARIAN/VEGAN,
  just leave out the Parmesan
✳ FAMILY-FRIENDLY,
  just leave out the salt

Ingredients

1 tablespoon olive oil
1 onion, diced
2 garlic cloves, finely chopped
1 teaspoon paprika
1 teaspoon dried oregano
2 red peppers, cored, deseeded
  and diced
100g/3½oz/1½ cups chestnut/
  cremini mushrooms, diced
100g/3½oz/½ cup frozen sweetcorn
2 x 400g/14oz can of chopped
  tomatoes
2 x 400g/14oz can of green lentils,
  drained
250g/9oz whole-wheat spaghetti
A few parsley sprigs, leaves chopped
Salt
Parmesan cheese, grated, to serve

1 Heat the oil in a frying pan over a low heat. Add the onion and a pinch of salt and cook for 3–4 minutes. Add the garlic along with the paprika and oregano. Cook for 2 minutes.

2 Add the red peppers and mushrooms to the pan, followed by the sweetcorn. Cook for 2–3 minutes. Add the tomatoes and lentils and simmer for 15–20 minutes.

3 Meanwhile, cook the spaghetti as per the packet instructions.

4 Divide the spaghetti between 2 plates and top with a portion of the bolognese. Sprinkle over the parsley and serve with a dusting of Parmesan.

>> **MIX IT UP:**
✳ Obviously, if you're looking for a meatier version, minced/ground beef or pork work well instead of the lentils (or for my favourite, use a combination of both).
✳ Use up any leftover veg you have, such as carrots and courgettes/zucchini.
✳ Try experimenting with different pulses too, such as kidney beans and borlotti beans, both of which would be lovely in this dish.

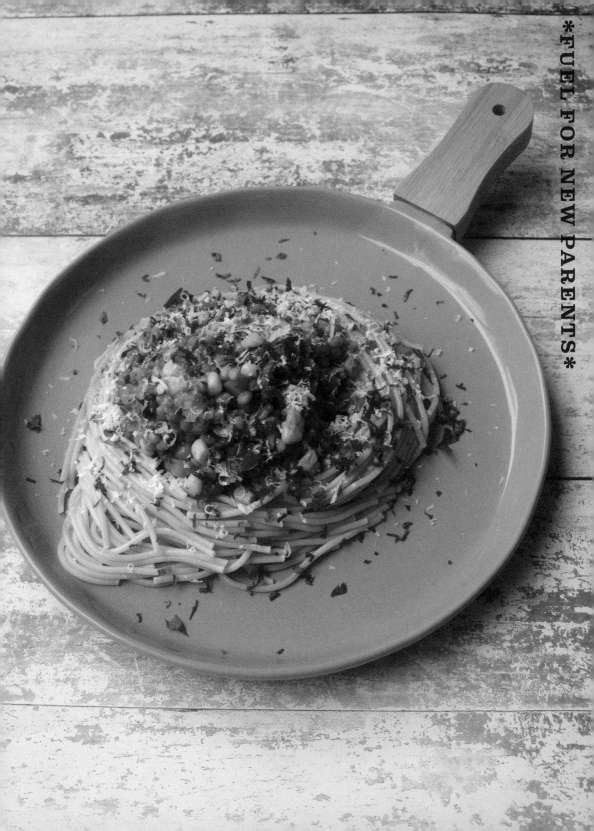

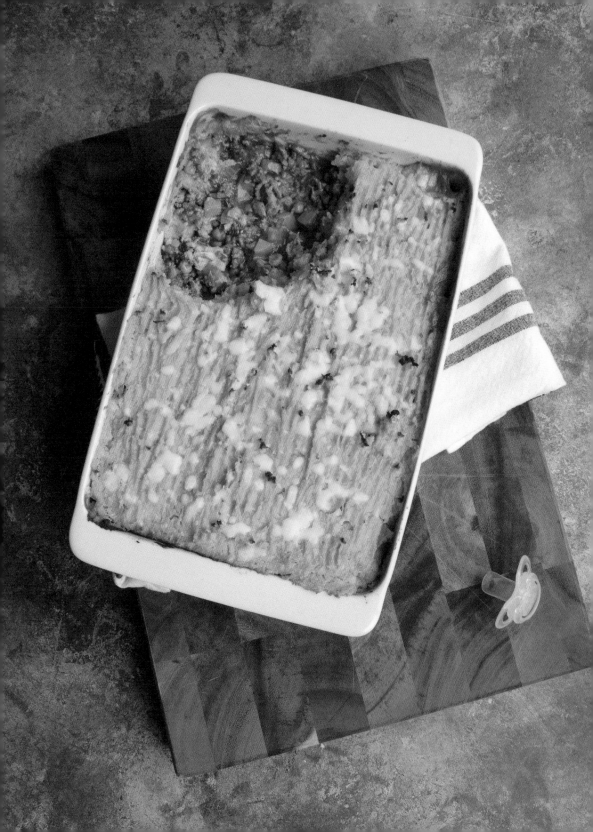

Cheesy Sweet Potato Shepherd's Pie

This is one of the best one-handed meals around. Make a big dish, then save portions in the freezer for when you need it most! Add some lentils to the beef for extra energy.

SERVES 2, plus loads
for the freezer
Prep time: 15 minutes
Cook time: 50 minutes

✳ BATCH COOK ME!
✳ FAMILY-FRIENDLY,
   just leave out the salt and use
   baby-friendly stock

Ingredients

1kg/2lb 4oz sweet potatoes, sliced
1 teaspoon olive oil
750g/1lb 10oz minced/ground beef
1 onion, diced
2 garlic cloves, crushed
3 carrots, diced
2 courgettes/zucchini, diced
100g/3½oz/½ cup frozen peas
2 celery stalks, diced
400ml/14fl oz/1⅔ cups beef stock
1 tablespoon tomato purée/paste
1 x 400g/14oz can chopped tomatoes
1 teaspoon chopped rosemary, fresh
   or dried
1 teaspoon chopped thyme, fresh
   or dried
1 teaspoon chopped oregano, fresh
   or dried
50g/1¾ oz/⅓ cup plain/all-purpose
   white flour (or any gluten-free
   alternative)
100g/3½oz/¾ cup Cheddar, grated,
   plus more for top
Salt

1 Preheat the oven to 180°C/350°F/Gas 4.

2 Cook the sweet potatoes in a pan of lightly salted boiling water for 5−7 minutes until soft. Drain and leave to cool.

3 Heat the olive oil in a pan over a high heat. Add the minced/ground beef and cook for 2−3 minutes until nicely browned. Set aside.

4 Add the onion to the pan along with a pinch of salt and cook for 2−3 minutes. Add the garlic, carrots, courgettes/zucchini, peas and celery and cook for a further 5 minutes.

5 Make the sauce. Whisk together in a bowl the stock, tomato purée/paste, tomatoes, herbs and flour. Pour into the pan, adding the beef back in too. Cook for a further 10 minutes.

6 Meanwhile, mix together the grated Cheddar and sweet potatoes in a bowl and mash well. Pour the beef mixture into a large ovenproof dish and top with the sweet potato mash. Sprinkle a little more grated Cheddar over the top and bake for 20 minutes.

> > **MIX IT UP:**
> ✳ Add some root vegetables, such as parsnips and swedes.
> ✳ Swap the sweet potato mash for puréed cauliflower or celeriac.
> ✳ Swap the minced/ground beef for lamb or pork, or for a vegan option combine diced mushrooms and lentils.

Harissa Chicken, Chorizo, Sweet Potato, Lentil and Vegetable One-Pot

A hodgepodge of a dish and one that's great for using up whatever is in the refrigerator. This is comforting food to fill up new parents and provide an energy boost to see them through the long nights!

SERVES 2
Prep time: 15 minutes
Cook time: 40 minutes

✳ BATCH COOK ME!

Ingredients

1 tablespoon olive oil
2 chicken breasts, diced into 2cm/1in cubes
200g/7oz chorizo, sliced
1 onion, diced
3 sweet potatoes, diced
3 carrots, diced
1 x 400g/14oz can of chopped tomatoes
2 teaspoons harissa paste
300ml/10½fl oz/scant 1¼ cups chicken stock
1 x 400g/14oz can of green lentils, drained
50g/1¾oz/1 cup kale, tough stalks removed, roughly chopped
Salt
4 tablespoons Greek yogurt (or a plant-based alternative), to serve
A few fresh parsley leaves, chopped, to serve

1 Heat the olive oil in a large frying pan over a medium heat. Add the diced chicken and cook for 5 minutes. Add the chorizo and cook for another 5 minutes so the chicken takes on the flavour of the chorizo, then set aside.

2 Add the onion to the pan along with a pinch of salt and cook for 2–3 minutes. Add the sweet potatoes and carrots and cook for a further 2–3 minutes.

3 Add the tomatoes, harissa paste, chicken and chorizo, and stock and mix well. Bring to the boil, then reduce the heat and simmer for 20 minutes.

4 Add the lentils and kale and cook for a further 2–3 minutes.

5 Serve with Greek yogurt and fresh parsley on top.

>> **MIX IT UP:**
✳ Swap the chorizo and chicken for some sliced portobello mushrooms and broccoli.
✳ For less heat swap the harissa paste for tomato purée/paste.
✳ Serve with some brown rice for extra carbs.

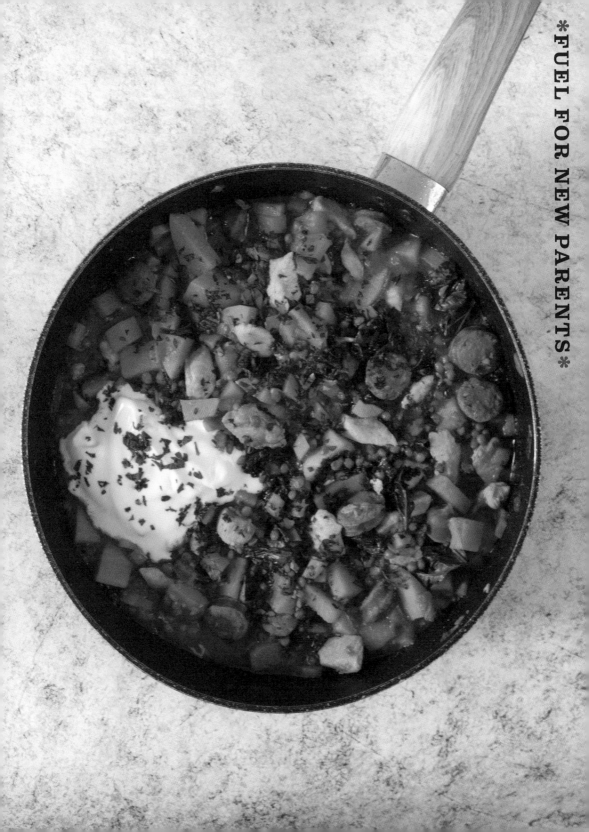

Cumin Chicken Broth with Olives, Brown Rice and Chickpeas

A comforting broth that's full of strong flavours. This is a great dish to make ahead, then just reheat when needed.

SERVES 2, plus plenty
   for the freezer
Prep time: 10 minutes
Cook time: 35 minutes

✳ BATCH COOK ME!
✳ FAMILY-FRIENDLY, just chop
   and crush the chickpeas/olives
   for baby

Ingredients

2 tablespoons olive oil
2 chicken breasts, diced into 2cm/
   1in cubes
1 onion, diced
1 teaspoon ground cumin
100g/3½oz/1 cup pitted green
   olives, halved
300g/10½oz/1½ cups brown rice
700–800ml/24–28fl oz/3–3½ cups
   chicken stock
1 x 400g/14oz can of chickpeas/
   garbanzo beans, drained
Zest of 1 lemon
A few parsley sprigs, leaves chopped
Salt

1 Heat a tablespoon of oil in a pan over a medium heat. Add the chicken, season and cook for 7–8 minutes. Set aside.

2 Heat another tablespoon of oil in the pan. Add the onion and cumin, season and cook for 3–4 minutes. Add the olives followed by the rice, stirring well to ensure the rice is coated with the flavours of the pan.

3 Pour in the stock and add the cooked chicken back in. Bring to the boil then reduce the heat and simmer for around 20 minutes, or until the rice is cooked. You want some liquid in the pot at the end, so add more stock if necessary as you go. Ensure the pan is covered or the rice won't cook quickly.

4 Add the chickpeas/garbanzo beans and cook for another minute.

5 Ladle out the broth into 2 bowls and sprinkle with lemon zest and some chopped parsley.

>> **MIX IT UP:**
✳ Swap the chicken for lamb or diced butternut squash.
✳ Replace the rice with couscous, pearl barley or buckwheat.

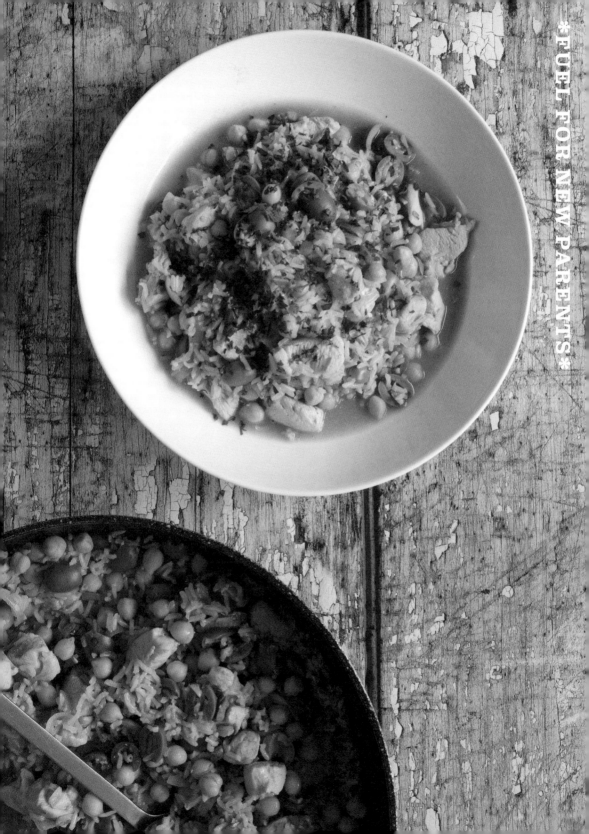

>> **MIX IT UP:**
✳ Try crumbling some paneer on top of the biryani while it's cooking for extra calcium.
✳ Combine half a teaspoon of each of the spices with a splash of oil and use it as a marinade for the salmon, or alternatively use chicken or lamb, or an entire roasted cauliflower for a vegan option.

Salmon Biryani

You can pack lots of spices and veg into this dish. It's a delicious and easy-to-make fakeaway to reward yourself at the end of a long day.

SERVES 2
Prep time: 15 minutes
Cook time: 30 minutes

✳ BATCH COOK ME!
✳ FAMILY-FRIENDLY,
   just leave out the salt and use
   baby-friendly stock

Ingredients

A knob of butter (or a vegan
   alternative)
1 onion, diced
2 garlic cloves, finely chopped
5cm/2in piece of fresh root ginger,
   peeled and grated
1 teaspoon ground coriander
1 teaspoon garam masala
1 teaspoon ground cumin
1 teaspoon ground turmeric
1 teaspoon mustard seeds
1 aubergine/eggplant, diced
1 carrot, diced
A few cauliflower florets
300g/10½oz/1½ cups long grain
   brown rice
600ml/21fl oz/2½ cups vegetable stock
1 teaspoon tomato purée/paste
12 new potatoes
100g/3½oz/½ cup frozen peas
2 salmon fillets, about 150g/5½oz each
Large handful of spinach, chopped
1 spring onion/scallion, chopped
A few coriander/cilantro sprigs, leaves
   chopped
Salt

1 Preheat the oven to 180°C/350°F/Gas 4.

2 Melt the butter in a saucepan over a medium heat. Add the onion along with a pinch of salt and cook for 2–3 minutes. Add the garlic, ginger and spices, then stir well so they coat the diced onion.

3 Add the aubergine/eggplant, carrot and cauliflower florets. Pour the rice into the pan along with the stock and stir in the tomato purée/paste. Bring to the boil, mix well, then reduce the heat to a simmer. Add the potatoes and stir in the peas. Cover the pan and cook for around 20 minutes. If the pan gets too dry, add some more stock.

4 While the biryani is cooking, place the salmon fillets in an ovenproof dish, season and bake for 10 minutes. Remove and keep warm.

5 When almost all of the liquid has been absorbed in the biryani pan and the rice is cooked, add the spinach and stir it in, allowing it to wilt.

6 Flake the salmon into chunks and place on top of the biryani. Finally, sprinkle over the chopped spring onion/scallion and coriander/cilantro and serve.

Roasted Salmon, Spiced Chickpeas and Vegetables

This is a quick and versatile dish that brings together lots of superfoods. It's also one that lends itself to batch-cooking, so is great to make ahead. Simply freeze the chickpeas/garbanzo beans and vegetables and cook the salmon separately each time. Try experimenting with different vegetables too.

SERVES 2

Prep time: 10 minutes

Cook time: 25 minutes

* BATCH COOK ME!

* FAMILY-FRIENDLY,
   just use baby-friendly stock

Ingredients

1 lemon

2 salmon fillets, about 150g/5½oz
   each

1 tablespoon olive oil

1 onion, diced

2 garlic cloves, crushed

1 teaspoon ground cumin

2 courgettes/zucchini, diced

2 carrots, diced

2 red peppers, cored, deseeded and
   diced

100ml/3½fl oz/scant ½ cup
   vegetable stock

2 handfuls of spinach leaves, chopped

50ml/2fl oz/3 tablespoons full-fat/
   whole milk (or a plant-based
   alternative)

2 x 400g/14oz can of chickpeas/
   garbanzo beans, drained

A few chives, chopped

1 Preheat the oven to 180°C/350°F/Gas 4.

2 Cut 4 slices from the lemon and place on a baking sheet, then place the salmon fillets on top. Squeeze the remaining lemon juice over the salmon and bake for 10−12 minutes.

3 Heat the oil in a pan over a medium heat. Add the onion and cook for 2−3 minutes. Add the garlic and cumin, stir well and cook for another minute.

4 Add the courgettes/zucchini, carrots and peppers and cook for a few minutes, then pour in the stock and cook for 5 minutes.

5 Add the spinach and cook for a minute until it wilts. Stir in the milk and the chickpeas/garbanzo beans and cook for a further 2−3 minutes.

6 Divide the vegetables between 2 bowls and top with the salmon and some chopped chives before serving.

> > **MIX IT UP:**
> * Add some diced chorizo to the pan, swap the spinach for kale, the chickpeas/garbanzo beans for lentils and the salmon for cod or haddock.

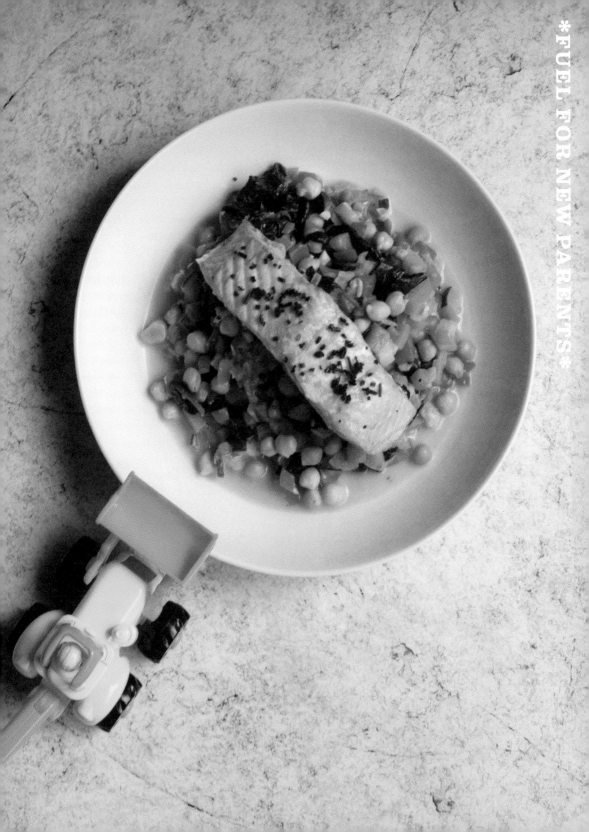

FUEL FOR NEW PARENTS

King Prawn and Extra Veg Aglio e Olio

There's nothing quite like a big bowl of garlicky, spicy pasta to look forward to at the end of the day. Add some chunky prawns/shrimp for a protein boost.

SERVES 2
Prep time: 10 minutes
Cook time: 15 minutes

✳ BATCH COOK ME!

Ingredients

250g/9oz whole-wheat spaghetti
2 tablespoons olive oil
1 onion, diced
4 garlic cloves, sliced
1 red chilli, deseeded and diced, or
    1 tablespoon dried chilli/hot
    pepper flakes
1 courgette/zucchini, diced
6–8 chestnut/cremini mushrooms,
    sliced
300g/10½oz raw peeled king
    prawns/jumbo shrimp
Juice of ½ lemon
30g/1oz/¼ cup Parmesan cheese
A few chives, chopped
Salt

1 Cook the spaghetti according to the packet instructions, then drain, reserving a few tablespoons of the pasta water.

2 Meanwhile, heat a tablespoon of the oil in a pan over a medium heat. Add the onion along with a pinch of salt and cook for 2–3 minutes. Add the garlic and chilli and cook for 2 minutes.

3 Add the courgette/zucchini and mushrooms along with 2 tablespoons of the retained pasta water. Cook for 3–4 minutes, then add the prawns/shrimp. Squeeze the lemon juice into the pan and cook until the prawns turn pink, about 3 minutes.

4 Add the cooked spaghetti to the pan along with the remaining olive oil and Parmesan. Mix everything together well, then divide between 2 plates. Top with chopped chives and serve.

> > **MIX IT UP:**
✳ Add some peas and roasted broccoli in place of the prawns/shrimp for a vegetarian aglio e olio.
✳ Swap the prawns/shrimp for some flaked salmon or sliced cooked chicken breast.

Chicken, Bacon, Leek and Mushroom Pie with Roasted Broccoli

A good old pie for new parents to devour. Who doesn't love puff pastry? And when it's on top of creamy chicken and veg, all the better. To save time, batch-cook the filling and top with pastry before cooking.

SERVES 2, plus lots for the freezer
Prep time: 15 minutes
Cook time: 50 minutes

✳ BATCH COOK ME!
✳ FAMILY-FRIENDLY,
    just leave out the salt and use
    baby-friendly stock

Ingredients

A knob of butter (or vegan alternative)
2 leeks, finely sliced
5–6 cloves of garlic, 2 crushed
1 teaspoon rosemary, fresh or dried
1 teaspoon thyme, fresh or dried
1 teaspoon sage leaves, fresh or dried
6–8 thick-cut bacon rashers/slices, diced
2–3 chicken breasts, cut into
    2cm/1in cubes
200ml/7fl oz/scant 1 cup chicken stock
50g/1¾ oz/⅓ cup plain/all-purpose
    white flour (or any gluten-free
    alternative)
200ml/7fl oz/scant 1 cup single
    cream (or a plant-based alternative)
250g/9oz/3¾ cups chestnut/cremini
    mushrooms, thickly sliced
1 egg, whisked
500g/1lb 2oz ready-made puff
    pastry, rolled out
1 head of broccoli, broken into florets
1 tablespoon olive oil
Salt

1 Preheat the oven to 180°C/350°F/Gas 4.

2 Melt the butter in a frying pan over a low heat. Add the leeks along with a pinch of salt and cook for 3–4 minutes. Add the 2 crushed garlic cloves, rosemary, thyme, sage, bacon and chicken and cook for a further 5 minutes.

3 In a jug combine the stock, flour and cream. Add the mushrooms to the pan, then pour over the liquid. Bring to the boil then reduce the heat and simmer for 8–10 minutes.

4 Spoon the filling into a suitable ovenproof dish. Brush the rim of the dish with some of the whisked egg, then lay the puff pastry over, ensuring the dish is totally covered. Prick the pastry with a fork a few times to allow the air to escape while it's cooking, then brush the top of the pastry with the remaining egg. Sprinkle over some salt and bake for 20–25 minutes until the pastry turns brown and crispy.

5 Place the broccoli in a baking pan with the remaining garlic. Drizzle over the olive oil, add a pinch of salt and roast for 20 minutes alongside the pie.

> > **MIX IT UP:**
> ✳ Swap the leeks for onion.
> ✳ Increase the amount of mushrooms and add peas and carrots for a veggie option.
> ✳ If you don't want to cook the broccoli separately, just add it to the pie.

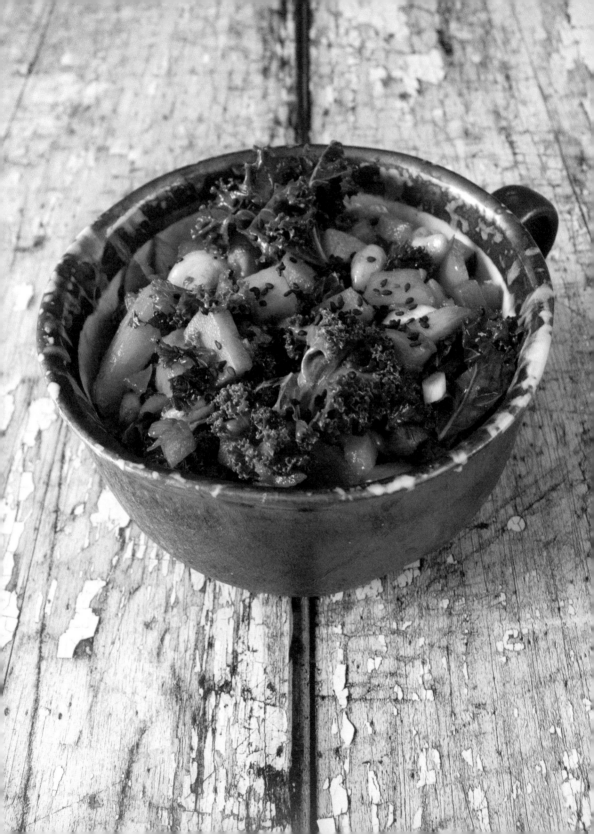

Sweet Potato, Pepper and Kale Stir-Fry

A very quick stir-fry dish using highly nutritious sweet potatoes and kale. Another energy-boosting meal to get you through those sleepless nights.

SERVES 2
Prep time: 10 minutes
Cook time: 25 minutes

* VEGETARIAN/VEGAN, if using maple syrup instead of honey

Ingredients

50g/1¾oz/⅓ cup cashew nuts

2 tablespoons vegetable oil

3 sweet potatoes, peeled and diced

1 shallot, diced

2 garlic cloves, crushed

5cm/2in piece of fresh root ginger, peeled and grated

1 red pepper, cored, deseeded and diced

4 tablespoons soy sauce

1 tablespoon sesame oil

1 teaspoon honey

1 teaspoon sriracha

1 teaspoon rice wine vinegar or white wine vinegar

3 large handfuls of kale, tough stalks removed, roughly chopped

2 tablespoons sesame seeds

2 spring onions/scallions, chopped

1 In a hot frying pan over a medium heat, dry-fry the cashew nuts for 3–4 minutes, then set aside.

2 Heat a tablespoon of the vegetable oil in a pan over a medium heat. Add the sweet potatoes, season with a pinch of salt and cook for 5–7 minutes, turning frequently. Remove and place on paper towels.

3 Heat another tablespoon of the vegetable oil in the pan. Add the shallot and cook for 2–3 minutes. Add the garlic and ginger and cook for 1 minute. Add the pepper and cook for another 2–3 minutes.

4 In a separate bowl, combine the soy sauce, sesame oil, honey, sriracha and vinegar.

5 Add the kale, cashew nuts, sweet potato and sauce to the pan and cook for a final 3–4 minutes.

6 Divide between 2 bowls and sprinkle with the sesame seeds and chopped spring onions/scallions before serving.

> > **MIX IT UP:**
> * Serve over brown rice, swap the peppers for courgettes/zucchini, peas and carrots or swap the sweet potato for tofu.
> * Garnish with some chopped fresh chillies.

Chilli Con Carne with Avocado and Brown Rice

You can't beat a good chilli con carne. It's a dish that lends itself well to batch-cooking, so it's perfect for new parents. Topping it with some avocado instead of sour cream also really increases the nutrient content. Try any leftovers on toast the next day – it's my guilty pleasure!

SERVES 2, plus some for the freezer
Prep time: 10 minutes
Cook time: 40 minutes

✳ BATCH COOK ME!
✳ FAMILY-FRIENDLY, just dial down the heat, leave out the salt and use baby-friendly stock

Ingredients

2 tablespoons olive oil
400g/14oz minced/ground beef
1 onion, diced
3 garlic cloves, crushed
½ teaspoon cayenne pepper (or more to increase the heat)
½ teaspoon paprika
½ teaspoon ground cumin
2 red peppers, cored, deseeded and diced
2 x 400g/14oz cans of chopped tomatoes
2 teaspoons tomato purée/paste
100ml/3½fl oz/scant ½ cup beef stock
250g/9oz/1 cup brown rice
Salt
2 avocados, peeled and destoned
Juice of ½ lime
2 x 400g/14oz cans of kidney beans, drained

1 Heat the oil in a pan over a high heat. Add the minced/ground beef and cook for a few minutes until nicely browned. Set aside.

2 Add the onion to the pan and cook for a few minutes before adding the garlic, cayenne pepper, paprika and cumin. Stir well so that the spices mix with the onions.

3 Add the beef back in, followed by the peppers and cook for 2 minutes before adding the tomatoes, tomato purée/paste and beef stock. Turn the heat down and allow to bubble away for 30 minutes or so.

4 Meanwhile, cook the rice as per the packet instructions.

5 Mash the avocados and mix with the lime juice.

6 When the sauce in the chilli has reduced right down, stir in the kidney beans and cook for 2 more minutes.

7 Serve with the rice and avocado on top.

> **MIX IT UP:**
✳ Try homemade hummus or baba ganoush on top of the chilli instead of avocado.
✳ Swap the beef out for 500g/1lb 2oz/2½ cups cooked lentils and/or chickpeas/garbanzo beans.

Turmeric-and-Tahini-Roasted Whole Cauliflower with Harissa Ratatouille and Buckwheat

A vegan showstopper! And a real marriage of flavours between the slightly spicy harissa ratatouille and the tangy turmeric-and-tahini-roasted cauliflower. You can either bake the cauliflower whole like in this recipe or use the marinade for basting cauliflower steaks. This dish is a shot in the arm for when tiredness hits.

SERVES 2

Prep time: 10 minutes
Cook time: 25 minutes

* VEGAN/VEGETARIAN

Ingredients

200g/7oz /generous 1 cup
   buckwheat
500ml/17fl oz/2 cups vegetable
   stock
1 teaspoon ground turmeric
2 tablespoons tahini
Juice of ½ lemon
3 tablespoons olive oil
1 head of cauliflower, base and leaves
   removed
1 shallot, diced
1 courgette/zucchini, diced
1 aubergine/eggplant, diced
1 red pepper, cored, deseeded and
   diced
1 x 400g/14oz can of chopped
   tomatoes
1 teaspoon harissa paste
A few parsley sprigs, leaves chopped
Salt

1 Preheat the oven to 180°C/350°F/Gas 4.

2 Rinse the buckwheat well and place in a saucepan over a medium heat. Pour over the vegetable stock. Bring to the boil, then reduce the heat and simmer for 15 minutes. Remove from the heat and keep covered for 10 minutes, then fluff up with a fork.

3 In a bowl, mix together the turmeric, tahini, lemon juice and 2 tablespoons of olive oil. Place the cauliflower in an ovenproof baking dish and spoon the mixture over the cauliflower, ensuring it is totally covered. Roast for 20 minutes.

4 For the ratatouille, heat a tablespoon of oil in a pan over a medium heat. Add the shallot along with a pinch of salt and cook for 2–3 minutes. Add the courgette/zucchini, aubergine/eggplant and pepper. Pour in the tomatoes and mix in the harissa, then cook for 10 minutes or so until most of the liquid has reduced.

5 Remove the cauliflower from the oven and either cut into steaks or place whole on top of the ratatouille and buckwheat. Finally, garnish with the chopped parsley.

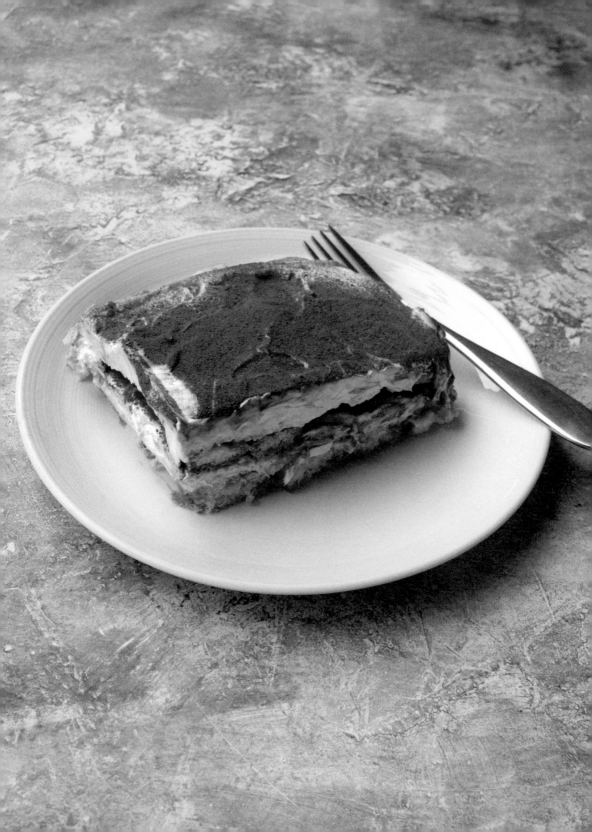

Tiramisu

Shortly after we came home from hospital with our first son, my wife informed me she would like to be left alone in bed with a tray of tiramisu and a fork. I duly obliged and it became a regular in the refrigerator for when she needed something sweet while feeding.

SERVES 1 (!)
Prep time: 15 minutes, plus
2 hours chilling time

Ingredients
500g/1lb 2oz mascarpone cheese
2 drops of vanilla essence/extract
50g/1¾oz caster/granulated sugar
2 eggs
1 packet of sponge fingers (around
30–40 sponge fingers)
250ml/9fl oz/1 cup strong coffee
4 tablespoons cocoa or hot chocolate
powder

1 In a large bowl, mix together the mascarpone, vanilla and sugar using a wooden spoon. Separate the eggs into whites and yolks then add the yolks to the bowl and mix well.

2 In a separate bowl, whisk the egg whites until stiff peaks form. Gently fold the egg whites into the mascarpone until mixed in.

3 Line the base of a dish measuring around 30cm x 20cm/12in x 8in with a layer of sponge fingers. Spoon a little coffee over the sponge fingers. You want to wet each one, but not soak them.

4 Spread half the mascarpone mixture over the sponge fingers, then sprinkle over half the cocoa or hot chocolate powder.

5 Add another layer of sponge fingers and repeat steps 3–4.

6 Refrigerate for at least 2 hours before eating.

>> **MIX IT UP:**
* Stir some fresh berries, pomegranate or lemon zest into the mascarpone mixture – or add some chocolate chips for an extra sweet boost.

Speedy Chocolate and Pomegranate Mousse

This chocolate mousse is delicious and only takes 10 minutes to make. When one of you is awake for a feed in the wee hours, tuck into this bad boy and treat yourself. Just make sure you make more if you take the last one from the fridge!

SERVES 4

Prep time: 10 minutes,
 plus 1–2 hours chilling time

Cook time: 5 minutes

Ingredients

150g/5½oz of milk or dark chocolate

20g/¾oz butter

3 eggs

1 tablespoon caster/granulated sugar

Seeds of 1 pomegranate

1 Bring a saucepan of water to the boil and place a heatproof bowl over it, making sure the bottom of the bowl doesn't touch the water. Break up the chocolate into the bowl and add the butter, stirring them together when they begin to melt. When melted completely, remove the bowl and leave to cool.

2 Separate the eggs. Add the egg yolks to the cooled chocolate and mix well. In a separate bowl, whisk the egg whites and sugar for 2–3 minutes until peaks are formed. Fold the egg whites into the chocolate, then mix in half the pomegranate seeds.

3 Spoon the mixture into 4 ramekins or bowls, cover and refrigerate for 1–2 hours. Serve with a spoonful of pomegranate seeds on top.

>> **MIX IT UP:**
* Add your favourite berries to the chocolate instead of the pomegranate.
* Serve with some whipped cream or ice cream to make it truly decadent.

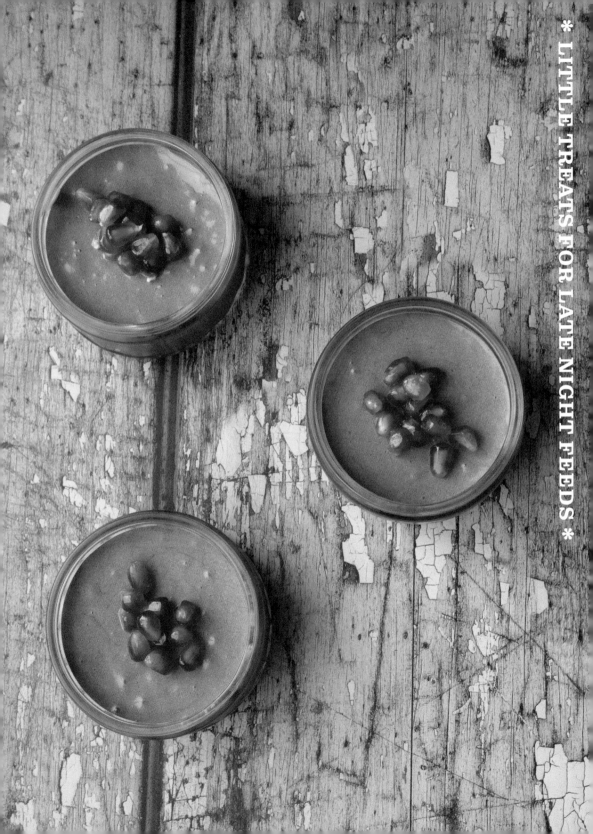

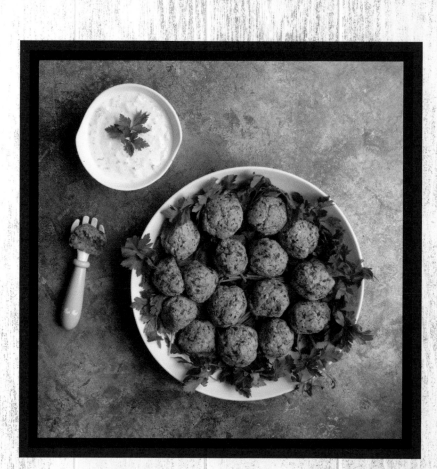

CHAPTER 5:
Baby's First Bites
(around 6 months onwards)

Starting Your Weaning Journey

Now the real fun begins! Starting your baby on their food journey is, in my opinion, an honour and something that should be fun for both parents and baby. Sure, there are times when it can be stressful or scary but try to embrace the mess and chaos. See this time as a great opportunity to experiment and explore different tastes with your baby. Have patience and relax. Don't drown in a world of steaming and puréeing every food under the sun. Try to see weaning as another time to further connect with your baby. Above all, remember that learning to eat is a skill, unlike anything baby has ever done before, and like all skills, it takes practice.

This chapter will give you a few ideas on different purées to give to baby in those first weeks of weaning after they have tried individual flavours and been exposed to different allergens. Then we'll move on to some weaning breakfast ideas and soft-textured foods full of different flavours perfect for the first few months. There are also finger foods perfect for batch-cooking that are tasty for the whole family.

Signs baby is ready

Your baby should be ready to start eating foods by the time they are 6 months old. In some cases, babies can be ready to try small amounts of purées from 4 or 5 months but please don't try to wean until your baby is ready. Different babies are ready at different times. Signs that they are ready include:

✳ Baby can sit comfortably without falling over and can hold their head steady. If they can't, they are not ready to wean.

✳ Hand, eye and mouth coordination. Baby can identify an object, pick it up and put it in their mouth. They are ready to start picking up finger food.

✳ Baby is curious about food. For the first few months of life, baby pays no attention to the fact that you are eating in front of them. When they suddenly begin to take an interest in what you are doing, and assuming the above points are also met, they are ready.

If you think your baby is ready and you start to feed them but they continually push the food out with their tongue, stop. Your baby is not ready.

Different approaches

There are many different approaches to weaning and none are better or worse than another. You know your baby best, so make the decision that's right for you. Some parents prefer to make purées and mashed foods to feed to baby, some prefer to make finger food, and some prefer to make baby-friendly meals and just leave baby to eat by themselves (known as baby-led weaning). Some choose to do all of the above. For my two children, my wife and I combined all approaches. We fed our children homemade purées of the dishes we were eating, made some meals just for baby and also made finger food to complement each meal. We fed them up until around nine months, at which point we encouraged them to spoon in foods by themselves – with varying degrees of success! This chapter follows the same approach, but again, you know what is best for your baby.

Kit

You could spend thousands on getting ready to wean your baby, but there are really only a few things you need. A highchair, bibs, plastic or rubber spoons, bowls and plates are essential. Invest in some ice-cube trays for freezing purées (and a few larger ice-cube trays for bigger portions) and some different-sized air-tight containers for the fridge so you're not making everything from scratch each day. You'll need a steamer for when you first start making vegetable purées and you can either buy one for this purpose or just steam the vegetables in a colander over boiling water. If you don't have one already, a blender or food processor that can work with small quantities is essential (I use a cheap hand blender). You really don't need anything else beyond that.

Embrace the mess

There is no getting away from it: weaning is pretty messy and both you and baby will probably need to change your outfits quite a few times a day! Make sure, if you can, that everywhere you feed baby is wipeable (no carpets!) and don't sit too close to your favourite possessions (or complain if they get covered in food). Allowing your baby to make as much mess as they want is really important. You want to teach baby to explore the tastes, smells and textures of foods because mealtimes for them are an extra sensory experience. If you tidy during a meal or try to clean them while they're eating, you are teaching them that what they're doing is wrong. Embrace the mess!

First foods (around 6 months)

Go slow at the start. Early-stage weaning is all about getting baby used to the new routine and the whole process of eating food. It's not about trying to get lots of different nutrients in. Up until this point, the only tastes that baby has ever had have been either breast or formula milk, both of which are sweet, meaning that baby is already predisposed to sweet tastes. It's therefore important to start weaning with tastes of bitter single vegetable purées such as broccoli, kale, aubergine/eggplant, cauliflower, green beans, courgettes/zucchini, peppers and so on. You can also try carrots, sweet potato, parsnips, peppers and squash but as they are quite sweet vegetables make sure you start with the bitter ones first. Simply chop and steam each vegetable and then blend into a purée. Make your purées in batches, freeze them in ice-cube trays, then defrost when required. You can also start mixing different flavours together after baby has tried everything once. Baby does not need to eat three times a day, so start with feeding once or twice a day when you are both calm and have the time to spend together. For finger foods, start to give baby some steamed broccoli, parsnips, carrots, cauliflower and so on to play with.

Introducing allergens

After you've spent around 10–14 days introducing the above vegetables to baby (and having a play around mixing different vegetables together), it's time to spend a few weeks introducing, one by one, small quantities of food that could trigger allergic reactions. The main ones are cow's milk, eggs, gluten, tree nuts, seeds, soy, shellfish and fish.

Start introducing allergens when baby is feeling well, i.e. no temperature, coughs or colds. Introduce the allergen during the breakfast or lunch feed so you have a longer amount of time to ensure that there are no reactions and leave three days between introducing allergens. Once you know baby has not suffered an allergic reaction and can tolerate the specific allergen, begin to use it regularly in their meals so that they are regularly exposed to it.

>> **COW'S MILK:** Add a splash of milk to porridge or a vegetable purée or give baby a little Greek yogurt to try.

>> **EGGS:** Give baby diced hard-boiled egg, some scrambled eggs or vegetable muffins (as long as you have first exposed them to cow's milk successfully).

>> **GLUTEN:** Try some pasta, cereal or wholegrain bread.

>> **TREE NUTS:** Stir some nut butter into baby's morning porridge.

>> **SEEDS:** Add some crushed seeds to baby's morning porridge (after you've successfully introduced nuts and peanuts.)

>> **SOYA:** Make some tofu for baby and serve it as a finger food.

>> **SHELLFISH:** Dice a cooked prawn/shrimp for baby, then mix it into a purée or give a prawn/shrimp to eat as finger food.

>> **FISH:** Cook a salmon fillet and use it as finger food, then mix it into a purée or make fishcakes with it.

What am I looking for?

An allergic reaction could include wheezing and shortness of breath, itchy throat and tongue, an itchy rash, swollen lips and throat, a runny or blocked nose, a cough, diarrhoea and vomiting, and sore, red and itchy eyes. In some cases, it may lead to a severe allergic reaction, so **if you are in any doubt or you think your baby may have had an allergic reaction to a food group, seek medical advice.**

Modifying Recipes if my Child has an Egg, Gluten or Milk and Dairy Allergy

Allergies in very young children are becoming diagnosed earlier and earlier nowadays, and while not every recipe will remain completely accessible or easy to modify, there are a few swaps you can make so the dishes are suitable for your little ones. As a reminder, please ensure you have introduced the major allergens to your baby one-by-one in the early stages of your weaning journey. See above for more information.

>> **EGG SUBSTITUTES FOR BAKING**

Chia or Linseed/Flaxseed egg: 1 tablespoon of chia seeds mixed with 3 tablespoons of cooled, boiled water. Mix and leave the chia seed for 5 mins to set, or refrigerate the linseed/flaxseed for 15 mins to set.

Alternatives: 1 mashed banana, 60g apple purée, 60g Greek yogurt.

Above quantities are for 1 "egg".

>> MILK AND DAIRY SUBSTITUTES

Plant-based yogurts, butters, milks and cheeses are all readily available and can be substituted in any recipe in this book. Please consult your doctor and read labels carefully as some should not be given to under-1s.

>> GLUTEN-FREE IDEAS

Swap in quinoa, gluten-free rice and pasta or potato variations when required throughout the book. Gluten-free flours such as almond, coconut and corn can be used in recipes and gluten-free baking powder is readily available.

Please ensure you consult your doctor first if you suspect your child has any allergies and create a comprehensive plan with them. Please be aware that the above substitutes will affect the nutritional content of each dish.

Beyond first foods (up to a year)

All in all, introducing first foods and different allergens will probably take you around 4 weeks, and then baby is really ready to start activating those tastebuds! Babies can eat most foods from six months onwards (see below for foods they can't eat), so now is the time to really have fun and start introducing lots of different foods as well as herbs and (gentle) spices. Don't be disheartened if baby rejects food at the start; it can take ten times or more for a food to be accepted. Equally, if baby loved something yesterday but won't eat it again today, don't worry, just keep going!

As long as there is no added salt in dishes, baby can also begin to eat the same food as the rest of the family, which is a huge timesaver. As always you know your baby best, but baby's food still needs to be either mashed, finely chopped, puréed or cut into finger food portions depending on how well they can swallow. From 7–9 months baby will begin to be able to swallow lumpier foods and will also eat finger foods relatively comfortably, so be careful but confident in progressively offering baby lumpier and thicker foods.

Apart from withholding salt and chilli, there is no reason to "dumb-down" dishes for baby, as exposing them to different tastes should be encouraged as much as possible.

Safety

Never, ever leave baby alone when they are eating. It is perfectly normal that baby will gag while they are eating foods early on and it's important that you let them do so; it's their gag reflex kicking in. You know they are gagging when their face turns red and they start to cough and splutter. They will then normally spit the food out and carry on as normal. It can be scary to witness as a parent, but the gag reflex is there to keep baby safe and it's best to not intervene. What's obviously not okay is if they start choking on food, turn blue, not red, and stay quiet as opposed to making lots of noise. If this happens, you need to **intervene as quickly as possible**. It's a good idea to either attend a course or read up on baby first aid before starting your weaning journey.

In terms of reheating food for baby, unless stated, always defrost frozen foods thoroughly in the fridge and then reheat until piping hot (then obviously stir and leave to cool before serving). Only reheat food once.

A typical day

A typical day in my house with an 8-month-old baby would look like this:

>> **BREAKFAST:** Either wholegrain porridge (with a few ground nuts, nut butter, seeds, grated or mashed fruits and vegetables mixed in, see page 156) or wholegrain bread with nut butter spread, scrambled eggs with herbs and cheese, or French toast on the weekends. A banana or breakfast muffin as finger food or breakfast on the go.

>> **LUNCH:** A mixture of leftover meals from the refrigerator or freezer, a slice of cheese, a sandwich cut into small pieces, a boiled egg, spreads and dips, finger foods, such as potato balls, fritters or frittatas, yogurt and fruit.

>> **DINNER:** A mashed or blended portion of what the rest of the family is eating, finger food, fruit and yogurt if not already eaten that day.

Foods to avoid

There are certain foods that are not recommended to give baby until they are a year old. These include honey and maple syrup, soft or unpasteurized cheeses, salty, processed and sugary foods. If you want to serve nuts, blend them in a food processor and sprinkle over porridge, cereal, etc. Consult your local health authority for a complete list.

SPOTLIGHT:

Five Introductory Purées

These purées are to get you started on your weaning journey. Spend a few days giving baby individual flavours and then begin combining different vegetables if you want. If you've frozen a lot of puréed vegetables, you can just chuck a few flavours together so baby can have a play around with different tastes. Think of it like a pic 'n' mix for baby! Adding different herbs and mild spices from 6 months is to be encouraged too. If the purées are running a little dry, add a splash of cooled boiled water, formula or breastmilk. If it's just a splash or two, and definitely mixed into food, cow's milk is also ok from 6 months onwards. (Please read the "introducing allergens" section on page 147 before using cow's milk).

∗ ALL OF THESE RECIPES MAKE ABOUT 12 ICE CUBES OF PURÉE ∗

∗ VEGAN / VEGETARIAN ∗

Asparagus, Pea and Mint

Ingredients
12–14 asparagus spears, woody ends removed ∗ 200g/7oz/1 cup peas ∗ A few mint sprigs

METHOD

1 Steam the asparagus until soft, about 5 minutes. Reserve a few for finger food, then add the rest to a food processor.

2 Add the peas and mint, then blend until smooth. Add a splash of liquid (see above), if needed, then leave to cool before serving.

Courgette, Green Bean and Basil

Ingredients
2 courgettes/zucchini, sliced into strips ∗ 100g /3½oz green beans, trimmed ∗ A few basil sprigs

METHOD

1 Steam the courgettes/zucchini and green beans until soft, about 5 minutes.

2 Reserve a few of each for finger food and add the rest to a food processor, along with the basil. Blend until smooth, adding a splash of liquid (see above), if needed, then leave to cool before serving.

Butternut Squash, Tomato and Parsley

Ingredients

1 butternut squash, peeled and thinly sliced
✳ 4 tomatoes ✳ A few parsley sprigs

METHOD

1 Steam the butternut squash until soft, about 10 minutes.

2 To peel the tomatoes, make a small cut through the skin on one side then plunge into boiling water for a minute or so. The skin should then peel away easily. Cut the tomatoes into slices and, reserving a few for finger food, add the rest to a food processor.

3 Reserve some of the steamed squash for finger food, and add the rest to the food processor. Add the parsley and blend until smooth. Add a splash of liquid (see above), if needed, then leave to cool before serving.

Leek, Spinach, Cauliflower and Oregano

Ingredients

1 leek, sliced lengthways ✳ 2 large handfuls of spinach leaves ✳ 1 head of cauliflower, cut into florets ✳ 1 tablespoon chopped oregano, or ½ tablespoon dried oregano

METHOD

1 Steam the leek until soft, about 10 minutes. When the leek is almost ready, add the spinach as it will steam very quickly. Place in a food processor.

2 Steam the cauliflower until soft, about 5 minutes. Reserve a few florets for finger food and add the rest to the food processor. Add the oregano and blend until smooth. Add a splash of liquid (see above), if needed, then leave to cool before serving.

Broccoli, Avocado and Carrot

Ingredients

1 head of broccoli, cut into florets ✳ 1 avocado, peeled, destoned and sliced ✳ 2–3 carrots, peeled and chopped ✳ 1 tablespoon lemon juice

METHOD

1 Steam the carrots and broccoli florets until soft, about 8 and 5 minutes, respectively. Reserve a few florets for finger food and place the rest in a food processor.

2 Reserve a few avocado slices for finger food and add the rest to the food processor. Add a splash of liquid (see above), if needed, then leave to cool before serving.

5 Purées for When You're Up and Running

When baby is older than 6 months and after a few weeks of experimenting with puréed vegetables and checking that your baby does not have a reaction to different allergens, you can start to add different food groups to the purées. Now is the time to introduce small protein and fibre-rich foods such as meat and fish, cheese, pulses and grains and so on. As before, if you need to add liquid, add a splash of cooled boiled water, formula, cow's milk or breastmilk.

✳ ALL OF THESE RECIPES MAKE ABOUT 12 ICE CUBES OF PURÉE ✳

Carrot, Cheddar, Chicken, Lentils and Rosemary

Ingredients
1 chicken breast, cut in half widthways ✳ Juice of ½ lemon ✳ 1 tablespoon fresh or dried rosemary ✳ 2 carrots, thinly sliced ✳ 1 x 400g/14oz can of green lentils, drained ✳ 50g/1¾oz/⅓ cup Cheddar cheese, grated

METHOD

1 Preheat the oven to 180°C/350°F/ Gas 4.

2 Place the chicken breast on a baking sheet. Squeeze over the lemon juice and sprinkle over the rosemary, then bake for 20 minutes.

3 Steam the carrots until soft, about 5 minutes.

4 Cut a few strips from the chicken to use as finger food and reserve a few carrot slices. Place the rest in a food processor along with the lentils and cheese and blend until smooth. Add a splash of liquid (see above), if needed, then leave to cool before serving.

Salmon, Pea, Sweet Potato and Cheddar

Ingredients

2 salmon fillets, about 150g/5½oz each, skin on ✳ Juice of ½ lemon ✳ 1 tablespoon chopped dill or 1½ teaspoons dried dill ✳ 2 sweet potatoes, cut into discs ✳ 100g/3½oz/½ cup peas ✳ 50g/1¾oz/⅓ cup Cheddar cheese, grated

METHOD

1 Preheat the oven to 180°C/350°F/Gas 4.

2 Place the salmon fillets on a baking sheet. Squeeze over the lemon juice and sprinkle over the dill, then bake for 12 minutes.

3 Meanwhile, cook the sweet potatoes in a pan of boiling water for 10 minutes until soft, then drain.

4 Remove the skin from the salmon and discard it. Cut off a few pieces from the salmon for finger food and place the rest in a food processor, along with the peas and cheese.

5 Reserve a few sweet potato discs for finger food and add the rest to the food processor. Blend until smooth. Add a splash of liquid (see above), if needed, then leave to cool before serving.

Cod, Courgette, Cannellini Bean and Oregano

Ingredients

2 cod fillets ✳ Juice of ½ lemon ✳ 1 tablespoon chopped oregano, or 1½ teaspoons dried oregano ✳ 2 courgettes/zucchini, sliced lengthways ✳ 1 x 400g/14oz can of cannellini beans, drained

METHOD

1 Preheat the oven to 180°C/350°F/Gas 4.

2 Place the cod fillets on a baking sheet. Squeeze over the lemon juice and sprinkle over the oregano, then cook for 12 minutes.

3 Meanwhile, steam the courgettes/zucchini until soft, about 5 minutes. Reserve a few pieces for finger food and add the rest to a food processor.

4 Cut off a few pieces from the cod for finger food, then add the rest to the food processor, along with the cannellini beans. Blend until smooth. Add a splash of liquid (see above) if needed, then leave to cool before serving.

Aubergine, Spring Onion, Red Pepper, Couscous and Thyme

Ingredients

200g/7oz/1⅓ cup couscous ✳ 200ml/7fl oz/scant 1 cup baby-friendly vegetable stock ✳ 1 tablespoon chopped thyme, or 1½ teaspoons dried thyme ✳ 1 aubergine/eggplant, peeled and sliced ✳ 1 red pepper, cored, deseeded and sliced ✳ 3–4 spring onions/scallions, trimmed and outer layer removed

METHOD

1 Prepare the couscous as per the packet instructions, using the vegetable stock and adding the thyme.

2 Steam the vegetables until soft, about 10 minutes. Reserve a few slices of aubergine/eggplant and red pepper for finger food and add the rest to a food processor along with the couscous. Blend until smooth, adding a splash of liquid (see above) if needed, then leave to cool before serving.

Broccoli, Mushroom, Lentils and Coriander

Ingredients

1 head of broccoli, cut into florets ✳ 6–8 chestnut mushrooms, trimmed ✳ 1 x 400g/14oz can of green lentils, drained ✳ A few coriander/cilantro sprigs

METHOD

1 Steam the mushrooms and broccoli until soft, about 8 minutes.

2 Reserve some broccoli florets for finger food. Place the remaining broccoli, mushrooms, lentils and coriander in a food processor and blend until smooth. Add a splash of liquid (see above) if needed, then leave to cool before serving.

How to Make your Porridge Sing

Breakfast is a great opportunity to get lots of nutrients into your baby. Porridge is such a wonderful dish to have each morning, as it's full of fantastic grains and will give baby lots of energy – which is especially helpful if they're burning the calories by crawling and learning to walk! As it's packed with fibre too, it's also good for their digestion. Here are a few ideas on how to add extra nutrients to porridge as well as playing around with the taste, texture and colour. You can make a batch and keep any leftover portions in the refrigerator for the working week. For the nuts, I tend to finely blend a mixture of 100g/3½oz/½ cup of cashew nuts, almonds and walnuts and keep in an airtight container until needed. To this day I still make this porridge for my children before they go to nursery, as I know it gives them the energy they need for the day!

SERVES 4–5 PORTIONS
Prep time: 10 minutes
Cook time: 5 minutes

✱ VEGAN/VEGETARIAN, if you
 use plant-based milk
✱ FAMILY-FRIENDLY

Ingredients

200g/7oz/2 cups rolled oats
600ml/21fl oz/2½ cups full-fat/whole
 milk, or a plant-based alternative, or
 a combination of both
4 bananas, mashed
2 carrots, grated
2 courgettes/zucchini, grated
2 apples, grated
4 tablespoons any nut butter (I prefer
 almond)
4 tablespoons very finely crushed
 mixed nuts
4 teaspoons chia seeds
2 teaspoons ground cinnamon

1 Place the oats in a saucepan over a medium heat and pour in the milk. Bring to a simmer and cook for around 5 minutes, stirring often, until most of the liquid has been absorbed.

2 Meanwhile, place the bananas, carrots, courgettes/zucchini and apples in a bowl. Add the nut butter and crushed nuts and mix well. Stir this into the porridge and mix well again. Top with the chia seeds and cinnamon.

3 Store any leftover porridge in airtight containers in the refrigerator for up to 5 days and simply reheat in a pan along with a splash of milk when needed.

> > **MIX IT UP:**
✱ There are lots of different ways to mix this up. Finely chop some blueberries or raspberries, grate some pear, experiment with different plant-based milks (I love using coconut milk), change the seeds you use (such as sesame or sunflower and crush them if necessary) and add different nut butters.

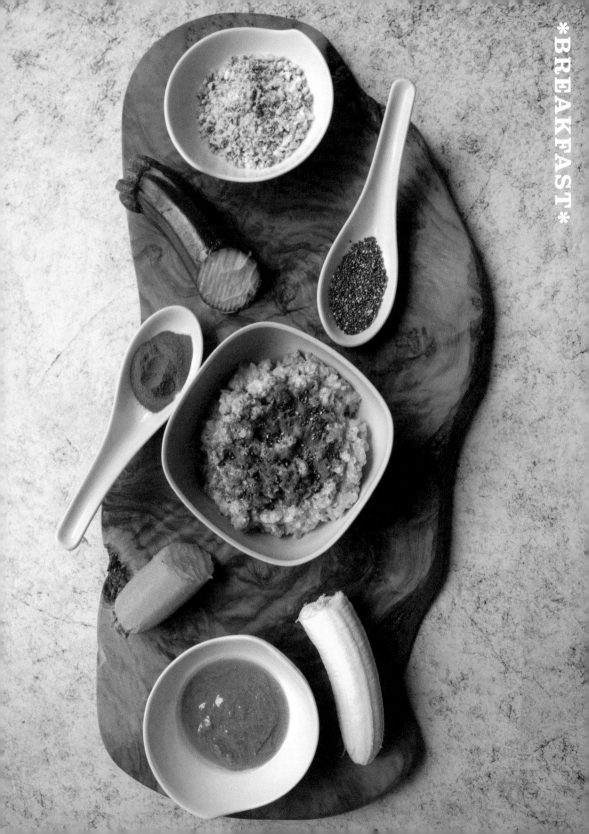

3 Easy Breakfast Muffin Ideas

Breakfast muffins are a great idea when you're on the go or in a rush. Each muffin is made from wholemeal/whole-wheat flour and contains no added sugar. Make a load for the freezer and simply take some out the night before for the morning. Alternatively, they're perfect for a mid-morning snack spread with butter.

✳ EACH RECIPE MAKES 12 ✳ PREP TIME: 10 MINUTES ✳
✳ COOK TIME: 20 MINUTES ✳ BATCH-COOK ME! ✳
✳ VEGETARIAN ✳ FAMILY-FRIENDLY ✳

Banana, Blueberry and Oat Muffins

Ingredients

Butter, for greasing

3 bananas, mashed

150g/5½oz/1½ cups blueberries

50g/1¾oz/½ cup rolled oats, plus
    2 tablespoons for the topping

1 egg

200ml/7fl oz/scant 1 cup full-fat/whole milk
    (or a plant-based alternative)

3 teaspoons olive oil

250g/9oz/1⅔ cups wholemeal /
    whole-wheat flour

2 teaspoons baking powder

> >> **MIX IT UP:**
> ✳ Mix and match any of these flavours. For example, apple would go really well with carrots and ginger.
> ✳ Add some chopped nuts and seeds and some raisins if your child is over one year old.

METHOD

1 Preheat the oven to 180°C/350°F/Gas 4 and grease a 12-hole muffin tray.

2 Place the bananas in a bowl with the blueberries and oats and mix together.

3 In a separate bowl, mix together the egg, milk and the oil.

4 Spoon the banana mixture into the egg mixture, then sift in the flour and baking powder. Mix everything together well, then spoon into the muffin tray. Sprinkle the top with oats and bake for 20 mins in the middle of the oven.

5 Leave to cool before removing from the tray. Either freeze or store in an airtight container for up to 2 days.

Apple, Pear and Cinnamon Muffins

Ingredients

Butter, for greasing

4 apples

2 pears

2 eggs

4 tablespoons Greek yogurt (or a plant-based alternative)

3 teaspoons olive oil

1 tablespoon ground cinnamon

250g/9oz/1⅔ cup wholemeal/whole-wheat flour

2 teaspoons baking powder

METHOD

1 Preheat the oven to 180°C/350°F/Gas 4 and grease a 12-hole muffin tray.

2 Grate the apples and pears, then squeeze the juice out with your hands (and drink it!).

3 In a large bowl, mix the fruit pulp with the eggs, yogurt, oil and cinnamon.

4 Sift in the flour and baking powder, mix well, then spoon into the muffin tray. Bake for 20 mins in the middle of the oven.

5 Leave to cool before removing from the tray. Either freeze or store in an airtight container for up to 2 days.

Carrot and Ginger Muffins

Ingredients

Butter, for greasing

3 carrots

5cm/2in piece of fresh root ginger, peeled

1 egg

4 tablespoons Greek yogurt (or a plant-based alternative)

3 teaspoons olive oil

250g/9oz/1⅔ cup wholemeal/whole-wheat flour

2 teaspoons baking powder

METHOD

1 Preheat the oven to 180°C/350°F/Gas 4 and grease a 12-hole muffin tray.

2 Grate the carrots and ginger, then squeeze the juice out with your hands (and drink it!).

3 In a large bowl, mix the carrot and ginger pulp with the egg, yogurt and oil.

4 Sift in the flour and baking powder, mix well, then spoon into the muffin tray. Bake for 20 mins in the middle of the oven.

5 Leave to cool before removing from the tray. Either freeze or store in an airtight container for up to 2 days.

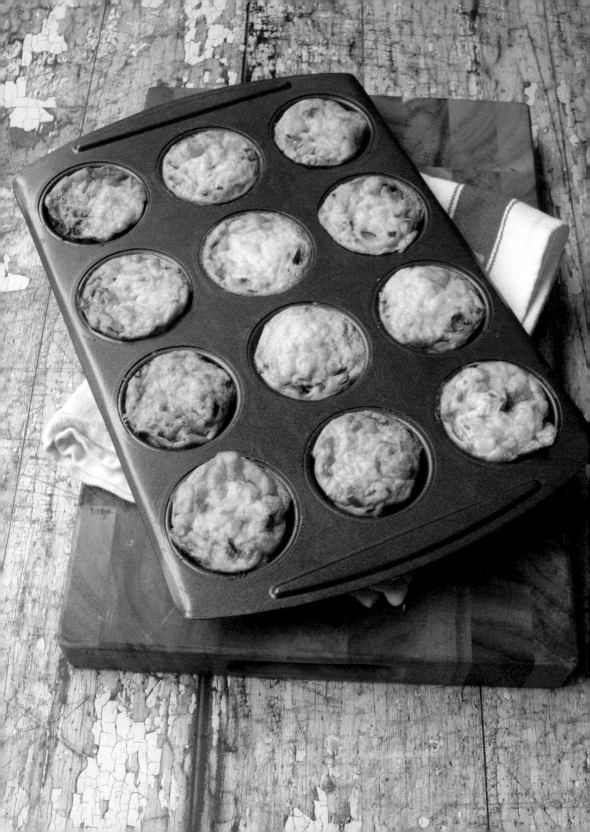

Egg and Vegetable Cups

If you're in need of a breakfast on the go or you're just really enjoying watching your baby get to grips with finger food, then give these a try. They're soft and springy, so perfect for tender gums. Make a batch and have breakfast sorted for the week.

MAKES 12
Prep time: 15 minutes
Cook time: 25 minutes

* BATCH COOK ME!
* VEGETARIAN
* FAMILY-FRIENDLY

Ingredients
Butter, for greasing
1 teaspoon olive oil
2 shallots, diced
A few thyme sprigs, leaves picked
1 courgette/zucchini, finely diced
1 red pepper, cored, deseeded and
    finely diced
1 green pepper, cored, deseeded and
    finely diced
4–5 asparagus spears, woody ends
    removed, finely chopped
6–8 chestnut mushrooms, finely
    chopped
Large handful of spinach leaves, finely
    chopped
8 eggs
50g/1¾oz/⅓ cup Cheddar cheese,
    grated

1 Preheat the oven to 160°C/325°F/Gas 3 and grease a 12-hole muffin tray.

2 Heat the oil in a frying pan over a medium heat. Add the shallots and thyme and cook for 2–3 minutes.

3 Add the courgette, peppers, asparagus and mushrooms and cook for 5 minutes until the peppers are soft. Add the spinach, stir, then remove the pan from the heat.

4 In a large bowl, whisk the eggs, then mix the cooked vegetables into the eggs. Spoon the mixture evenly into each muffin hole. Sprinkle a little Cheddar on top and bake for 15 minutes.

5 Leave to cool before removing from the tray. They will keep in an airtight container in the refrigerator for up to 3 days.

>> **MIX IT UP:**
* Dice up a little cooked sausage or bacon to stir in.
* Serve with some hot sauce for the adults.

Baked Sweet Potato Balls Three Ways

These not only combine lovely flavours, but baby will also love pulling them apart and investigating the different textures. Make in batches and freeze, then bake from frozen for about 20 minutes at 180ºC/350ºF/Gas 4 or until piping hot, whenever you need. Create golf-ball-sized for the adults or break up into smaller balls for baby.

* EACH RECIPE MAKES AROUND 16 BALLS *
* PREP TIME: 20 MINUTES * COOK TIME: 50–60 MINUTES *
* BATCH-COOK ME! *FAMILY-FRIENDLY *

Salmon, Cheese, Pea and Dill

Ingredients

3–4 large sweet potatoes, sliced * 1 lemon * 2 salmon fillets, about 150g/5½oz each, skin on * 100g/3½oz/½ cup peas * 50g/1¾oz/⅓ cup Cheddar cheese. grated * 1 tablespoon dried dill * 50g/1¾oz/½ cup Panko breadcrumbs * 1 egg * 3 tablespoons olive oil

METHOD

1 Preheat the oven to 180°C/350°F/Gas 4.

2 Cook the sweet potatoes in a pan of boiling water for 7–8 minutes. Drain, leave to cool, then mash.

3 Cut 4 slices from the lemon and lay them on a baking sheet. Place the salmon on top of the lemon slices and squeeze over the remaining lemon juice. Bake for 10 minutes in the oven.

4 Remove the skin from the salmon and discard. Place the salmon flesh in a food processor along with the peas, Cheddar, dill and breadcrumbs. Pulse briefly then transfer to a bowl and add the mashed sweet potato. Crack in the egg and mix everything together by hand. Shape into golf-ball-sized balls, then refrigerate for 30 minutes.

5 Spoon the olive oil onto a plate and roll each ball in the oil so it covers it thinly. Place the balls in a baking pan and bake for 40 minutes.

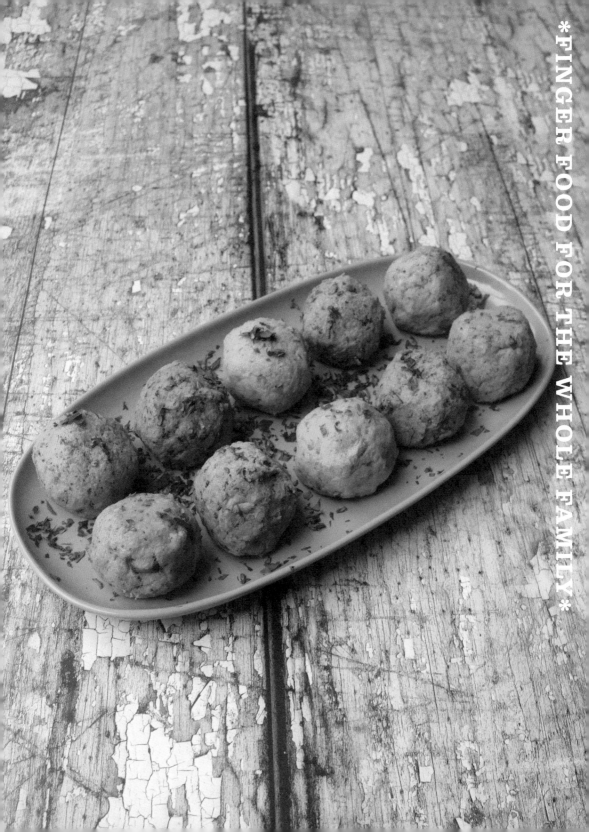

FINGER FOOD FOR THE WHOLE FAMILY

Chicken, Broccoli, Mushroom, Cheese and Rosemary

Ingredients

3–4 large sweet potatoes * 2 tablespoons olive oil * 1 chicken breast, cut into strips * 3–4 large chestnut mushrooms, diced *5–6 broccoli florets * 50g/1¾oz/⅓ cup Cheddar cheese, grated * 1 tablespoon dried rosemary * 50g/1¾oz/½ cup Panko breadcrumbs * 1 egg

METHOD

1 Heat the oven to 180°C/350°F/Gas 4.

2 Cook the sweet potatoes in a pan of boiling water for 7–8 minutes. Drain, leave to cool, then mash.

3 Heat a tablespoonful of the oil in a frying pan over a medium heat. Add the chicken and mushrooms and cook for 10 minutes.

4 Meanwhile, cook the broccoli in a pan of boiling water for 5 minutes. Drain and refresh under cold water.

5 Place the chicken and mushrooms in a food processor along with the broccoli, Cheddar, rosemary and breadcrumbs. Pulse briefly then transfer to a bowl and add the mashed sweet potato. Crack in the egg and mix everything together by hand. Shape into golf-ball-sized balls, then refrigerate for 30 minutes.

6 Spoon the remaining oil onto a plate and roll each ball in the oil so it covers it thinly. Place the balls in a baking pan and cook for 40 minutes.

Lentil, Spinach, Cheese and Parsley

Ingredients

3–4 large sweet potatoes, sliced * 2 large handfuls of spinach leaves, chopped * 1 x 400g/14oz can of green lentils, drained * 50g/1¾oz/⅓ cup Cheddar cheese, grated * 1 tablespoon dried parsley * 50g/1¾oz/½ cup Panko breadcrumbs * 1 egg * 4 tablespoons olive oil

METHOD

1 Follow steps 1 and 2 from the recipe above.

2 Place the spinach in a colander and pour hot water over it. Refresh under cold water, then press the water out.

3 Place the spinach in a food processor along with the lentils, Cheddar, parsley and breadcrumbs. Pulse briefly, then transfer to a bowl and add the mashed sweet potato. Crack in the egg and mix everything together by hand. Shape into golf-ball-sized balls. Refrigerate for 30 minutes.

4 Pour the oil on a plate. Roll each ball in the oil to thinly cover it. Bake the balls in a baking pan for 40 minutes.

Broccoli, Kale and Cheddar Wholemeal Mini Scones

These mini scones are perfect for a mid-morning or afternoon snack, for road trips, pram snacks or to complement a purée or two. They're packed full of complex carbs, calcium and folate, as well as other nutrients. This recipe makes about 48 mini scones to pop in the freezer; they defrost really quickly. I make these along with the veggie-packed muffins (see page 172) once a month, so I always have something to hand.

MAKES ABOUT 48 MINI SCONES

Prep time: 10 minutes
Cook time: 20 minutes

✱ BATCH COOK ME!
✱ VEGETARIAN
✱ FAMILY-FRIENDLY

Ingredients

Butter, for greasing

2 heads of broccoli, cut into florets

400g/14oz/2⅔ cups self-raising wholemeal/self-rising whole-wheat flour (or any alternative)

200g/7oz /¾ cup + 2 tablespoons butter (or a plant-based alternative)

200g/7oz/1½ cups Cheddar cheese, grated

3 large handfuls of kale, tough stalks removed, roughly chopped

5 tablespoons full-fat/whole milk (or a plant-based alternative)

1 Preheat the oven to 180°C/350°F/Gas 4 and grease a baking pan.

2 Cook the broccoli florets in boiling water for around 5 minutes. Drain, then finely chop.

3 In a bowl, combine the flour and butter with your fingers until the mixture resembles sand. Add the Cheddar, kale and broccoli and mix well. Add the milk, then mix well again.

4 Shape the mixture into small balls, place in the greased baking pan and bake for around 10−12 minutes. Remove and leave to cool.

> > **MIX IT UP:**
> ✱ Add some Parmesan or crumble in feta.
> ✱ Add cauliflower or leafy greens, such as cavolo nero/black kale or spinach (steam first to remove the water).
> ✱ Add herbs such as basil or oregano.

Three Easy and Nutritious Fish Spreads

Canned mackerel, sardines and tuna are not only cheap but a great way to introduce healthy fish into your baby's diet. But it can be hard to know how to serve them for baby. Making them into spreads is an easy and tasty solution. Add yogurt, egg, cheese or avocado to the spread for extra flavour and nutrients. Spread on thinly sliced bread, wraps or rice cakes, serve alongside some peeled and chopped vegetables, such as cucumber, or with cooked broccoli and carrot for dipping. They all last for 24–48 hours in the refrigerator.

* EACH RECIPE MAKES 2–3 PORTIONS,
OR ENOUGH FOR A SHARED LUNCH *
* PREP TIME: 5 MINUTES * COOK TIME (JUST THE EGG): 5 MINUTES *
* FAMILY-FRIENDLY *

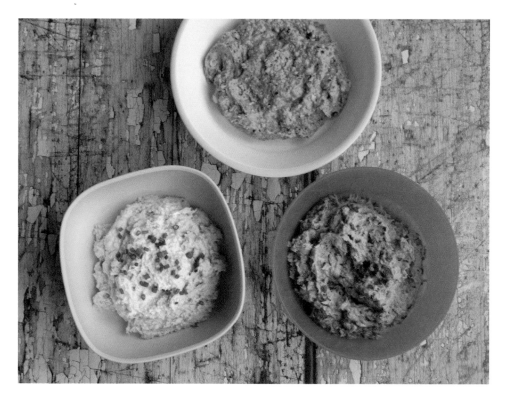

Mackerel, Chive and Greek Yogurt

Ingredients

2 smoked mackerel fillets, about 75–100g/2½–3½oz each, or 150–200g/5½–7oz canned mackerel, drained

2–3 tablespoons Greek yogurt (or a plant-based alternative)

Juice of ½ lemon

1–2 tablespoons Panko breadcrumbs (to thicken, if needed)

A few chives, chopped

METHOD

1 Remove the skin from the mackerel and place the flesh in a food processor along with the yogurt and lemon juice.

2 Blend until smooth, adding breadcrumbs, if required. Serve with a few chopped chives on top.

Sardines and Avocado

Ingredients

150–200g canned sardines, drained

1 avocado, peeled and destoned

Juice of ½ lemon

1–2 tablespoons Panko breadcrumbs (to thicken, if needed)

A few parsley sprigs, leaves chopped

METHOD

1 Place the sardines in a food processor along with the avocado and lemon juice.

2 Blend until smooth, adding breadcrumbs if required. Serve with chopped parsley on top.

> > **MIX IT UP:**
> ✳ Mix and match the ingredients in all three of these recipes.
> ✳ Add kale for extra nutrition.
> ✳ Swap the yogurt for cream cheese or a plant-based cream.

Tuna, Spinach, Cheese and Egg

Ingredients

1 egg

150–200g canned tuna, drained

20g/¾oz spinach leaves

20g/¾oz Cheddar cheese

1–2 tablespoons Panko breadcrumbs (to thicken, if needed)

METHOD

1 Cook the egg in a pan of boiling water for 5 minutes. Drain, then run under cold water. When cool enough to handle, peel and place in a food processor.

2 Add the tuna, spinach and Cheddar and blend until smooth, adding breadcrumbs, if required.

Spiced Courgette, Pea and Feta Fritters with Turmeric Yogurt

This is my favourite recipe in this chapter. These were such a hit with my second born; he ate nothing else for two days and would shout at me if we ran out. A great way of introducing different textures and spices to baby, these fritters go so well with the turmeric yogurt. Any leftovers will last 48 hours in the refrigerator.

MAKES 12
Prep time: 15 minutes
Cook time: 20 minutes

✳ VEGETARIAN
✳ FAMILY-FRIENDLY

Ingredients

100g/3½oz/½ cup frozen peas

2 courgettes/zucchini, grated

3–4 spring onions/scallions, finely chopped

2 garlic cloves, crushed

1 teaspoon ground cumin

1 teaspoon ground coriander

1½ teaspoons ground turmeric

2 eggs

100g/3½oz/⅔ cup plain/ all-purpose white flour (or any alternative)

1 teaspoon baking powder

Juice of ½ lemon

100g/3½oz/⅔ cup feta, crumbled

3–4 tablespoons vegetable oil, for frying

3 tablespoons Greek yogurt (or a plant-based alternative)

1 Place the peas in a bowl and pour hot water over them. Leave for 5 minutes, then drain and either pulse briefly in a food processor or crush slightly with a fork.

2 Place the grated courgettes/zucchini in a colander and squeeze out any excess water. In a bowl, mix with the peas. Add the spring onions/scallions and garlic.

3 Mix in the cumin, coriander and 1 teaspoon of the turmeric. Crack in the eggs and mix everything together with your hands. Sift in the flour and baking powder and mix into a batter. Add the lemon juice. It will be quite wet; don't worry! Finally, mix in the feta.

4 Heat half the vegetable oil in a wide frying pan over a medium heat. With your hands, shape a palm-sized portion ball of batter, then flatten slightly to a disc around 1cm/½in thick. Place in the frying pan. Repeat with the remaining mixture. You don't want to overcrowd the pan, so you may need to cook in batches and add a little more oil for each batch; I normally cook 4 at a time. Cook for 3–4 minutes, then flip them over and cook for a further 2 minutes. Remove and leave to cool on paper towels to absorb any excess oil.

5 Mix the yogurt in a bowl with the remaining turmeric. Serve alongside the cooled fritters.

>> **MIX IT UP:**
* Add some sweetcorn and grated carrot.
* Leave out the feta or replace with a milder grated cheese, if you prefer.
* Serve with a poached egg on top and some hot sauce for adults.

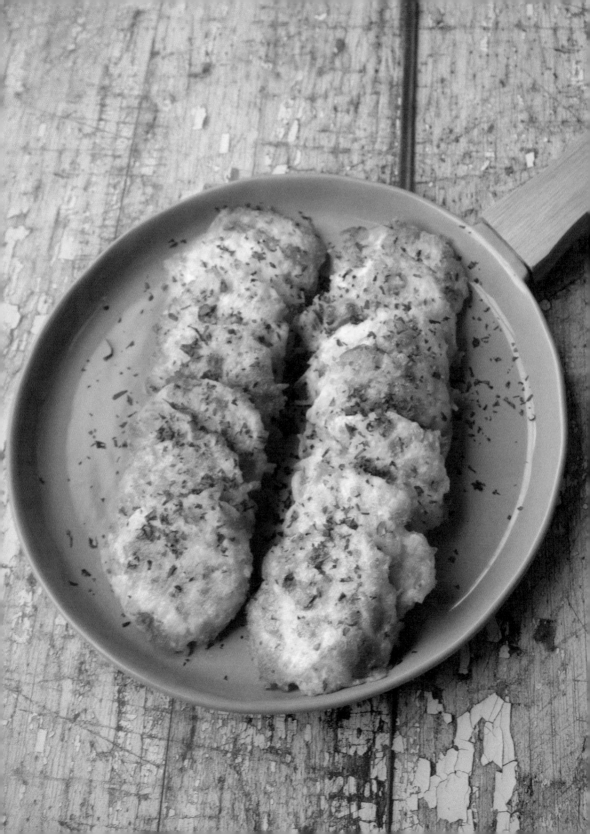

Potato and Cheese Rosti

Rostis are definitely a guilty pleasure in my house and both my wife and I find it hard to not eat about six of these each while feeding the little ones. These are ready in minutes and are a great finger food for baby. There's no need to cook the potato separately prior to making the rostis; because you're grating it, they'll cook in minutes.

MAKES ABOUT 24 ROSTIS

Prep time: 15 minutes
Cook time: 25 minutes

* ✱ BATCH COOK ME!
* ✱ VEGETARIAN
* ✱ FAMILY-FRIENDLY

Ingredients

5 large potatoes, grated
200g/7oz/1½ cups Cheddar cheese, grated
2 eggs, beaten
3 tablespoons plain/all-purpose white flour (or any alternative)
A knob of butter, for frying

1 Place the grated potatoes in a large bowl, then add the Cheddar and pour in the beaten eggs. Use your hands to mix everything together well. Sift in the flour and mix again. The mixture will be quite wet but don't worry.

2 Melt the butter in a frying pan over a medium heat. Using your hands, shape some of the mixture into a fist-sized disc about 1cm /½in thick and cook for 2–3 minutes per side so that the rostis get nice and crispy. Cook them in batches so you don't crowd the pan. You may need to add a little more butter with each batch. Remove from the pan and leave to cool on paper towels to absorb any excess oil.

3 Cut the rostis into thin strips to use as finger food for those under 9 months or so, or give whole to older babies or toddlers.

4 They'll keep for 48 hours in an airtight container in the refrigerator.

> > **MIX IT UP:**
> ✱ Add in some grated courgette/zucchini, carrot, frozen peas or sweetcorn for added nutrition.
> ✱ Add a can of tuna or some chopped cooked bacon too.

Wholemeal Veggie-Packed Cheese Muffins

I've made a batch of these every month since my eldest was 6 months old and I swear by them! There's always a load in our freezer. They are perfect for lunches, picnics and food on the go.

MAKES 12 MUFFINS OR 24 MINI MUFFINS

Prep time: 15 minutes
Cook time: 25 minutes

* BATCH COOK ME!
* VEGETARIAN
* FAMILY-FRIENDLY

Ingredients

Butter, for greasing
2 courgettes/zucchini, grated
2 carrots, grated
100g/3½oz/½ cup peas
100g/3½oz/¾ cup sweetcorn
2 tablespoons dried or fresh oregano
5 teaspoons Greek yogurt (or a plant-based alternative)
3 tablespoons olive oil
3 eggs, beaten
200g/7oz/1½ cups Cheddar cheese, grated
300g/10½oz/2 cups wholemeal/whole-wheat flour (or a gluten-free alternative)
3 teaspoons baking powder

1 Preheat the oven to 180°C/350°F/Gas 4 and grease a 12-hole muffin tray.

2 Squeeze excess water out of the courgettes/zucchini and carrots then place in a large bowl. Add the peas and sweetcorn along with the oregano, yogurt, oil, eggs and cheese. Mix well with your hands.

3 Sift in the flour and baking powder and mix again. You're looking for quite a sticky paste. Divide the mixture into the muffin holes.

4 Bake for 25 minutes. Remove and leave to cool before removing. If making mini muffins, cook for 12–15 minutes.

>> **MIX IT UP:**
* Literally any vegetable works well here, so feel free to experiment.

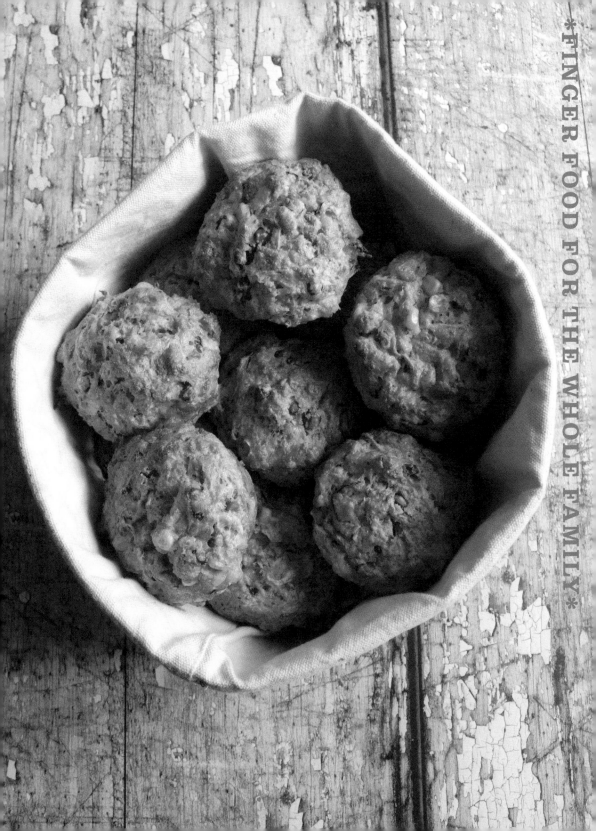

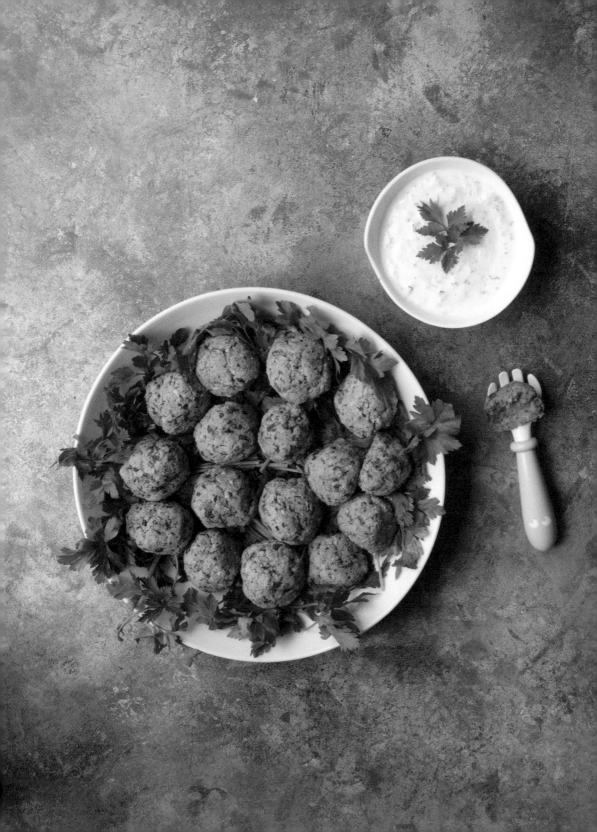

Chickpea and Pea Falafel with a Tzatziki Dip

These falafel are baked not fried and are a great way of introducing different textures and spices to baby. Dip them in some cool tzatziki and let baby make a mess! Stuff some falafel into a pitta with some greens, cucumber and tomatoes, all finished off with some tzatziki, for a quick and delicious adult lunch.

MAKES AROUND 20 FALAFEL

Prep time: 10 minutes
Cook time: 40 minutes

* BATCH COOK ME!
* VEGETARIAN/VEGAN, just use plant-based yogurt
* FAMILY-FRIENDLY

Ingredients

2 garlic cloves, crushed

1 shallot, diced

½ bunch of parsley

½ bunch of coriander/cilantro

Juice of ½ lemon

2 x 400g/14oz can of chickpeas/garbanzo beans, drained

100g/3½oz/½ cup peas

1 teaspoon ground cumin

1 teaspoon ground coriander

5 teaspoons plain/all-purpose white flour (or any alternative)

1 teaspoon baking powder

2–3 tablespoons olive oil

200g/7oz/scant 1 cup Greek yogurt (or a plant-based alternative)

¼ cucumber, peeled and finely grated

A few mint sprigs, leaves finely chopped

1 Preheat the oven to 180°C/350°F/Gas 4.

2 Place one of the garlic cloves and the shallot in a food processor along with the parsley and fresh coriander/cilantro. Squeeze in the lemon juice and add the chickpeas/garbanzo beans, peas, cumin, ground coriander, flour and baking powder. Pulse to a chunky consistency (not as smooth as a purée), then shape into golf-ball-sized balls.

3 Drizzle the olive oil onto a plate and roll each ball in the oil. Place the balls on a baking tray and bake for 40 minutes, turning once. Remove and leave to cool.

4 Meanwhile, to make the tzatziki, mix together the yogurt, cucumber, mint and remaining garlic clove.

>> **MIX IT UP:**
* Have a play with different ingredients. Some finely chopped nuts, different vegetables, such as sweetcorn and carrots, and additional pulses/legumes, such as broad beans and lentils, would work well.

>> **MIX IT UP:**
* Make these as you would any pizza, adding whatever toppings you want — just make sure they're all diced small enough for baby.
* Add some pineapple, shredded chicken, diced olives, bacon, minced/ground beef or prawns/shrimp.

Wholemeal Pitta Pizzas

Baby's first pizza! Baby will adore these little fingers of goodness, which will hopefully set them up for a lifetime love of pizza. These keep well in the refrigerator and because the cheese hardens up, they're easy to eat the next day too. If you have any of the veg mix left over, stir it through pasta for an additional dish. Make enough for you too and enjoy!

MAKES 4 PIZZAS

Prep time: 10 minutes
Cook time: 20 minutes

* VEGETARIAN
* FAMILY-FRIENDLY

Ingredients

1 tablespoon olive oil

2 shallots, finely diced

2 garlic cloves, finely chopped

1 red pepper, cored, deseeded and finely diced

1 green pepper, cored, deseeded and finely diced

1 courgette/zucchini, finely diced

3–4 chestnut mushrooms, finely diced

2 tablespoons tomato purée/paste

1 tablespoon oregano

4 wholemeal/whole-wheat pitta breads

200g/7oz /2 cups mozzarella, grated

1 Preheat the oven to 180°C/350°F/Gas 4.

2 Heat the oil in a pan over a medium heat. Add the shallots and garlic and cook for a couple of minutes. At 2-minute intervals add the peppers, then the courgette/zucchini and then the mushrooms.

3 Stir the tomato purée/paste and 2 tablespoons of water into the pan along with the oregano. Mix well and cook for a further 2 minutes, adding a little more water if the mixture runs dry.

4 Lay the pittas on a baking sheet and top with the cooked vegetables. Sprinkle over the grated mozzarella.

5 Bake for 6–8 minutes, or until the cheese has melted, then serve. For baby, leave to cool, then cut into finger-sized portions.

6 Any leftover pizzas will keep in the refrigerator for 2 days. (There won't be any leftovers.)

Arancini made from Leftover Risotto

Not only are arancini a delicious way of using up leftover risotto, they're also super quick to make and brilliant finger food for little hands. This recipe bakes the arancini rather than fries them. For risotto recipes see pages 70 and 190.

MAKES 18–20
Prep time: 10 minutes
Cook time: 20 minutes

✷ FAMILY-FRIENDLY

Ingredients

250–300g/9–10½oz leftover risotto rice (from the refrigerator)
50g/1¾oz /⅓ cup grated cheese (such as Cheddar, mozzarella or Gouda)
100g plain/all-purpose white flour (or any alternative)
3 eggs, beaten
200g/7oz/2 cups Panko breadcrumbs

1 The leftover risotto needs to be cold so if yours isn't, whack it in the refrigerator for an hour or so.

2 Preheat the oven to 180°C/350°F/Gas 4.

3 Place the risotto in a bowl and add the grated cheese. Mix well, then shape into golf-ball-sized balls.

4 In three separate bowls, place the flour, whisked eggs and breadcrumbs.

5 Dip and roll each ball first in the flour, then the egg and then the breadcrumbs. Place in an ovenproof dish.

6 Bake for around 15–20 minutes. For baby, leave to cool, then cut into quarters.

>> **MIX IT UP:**
✷ You can use any risotto you wish but if you are feeding this to a baby, make sure everything is chopped small enough.

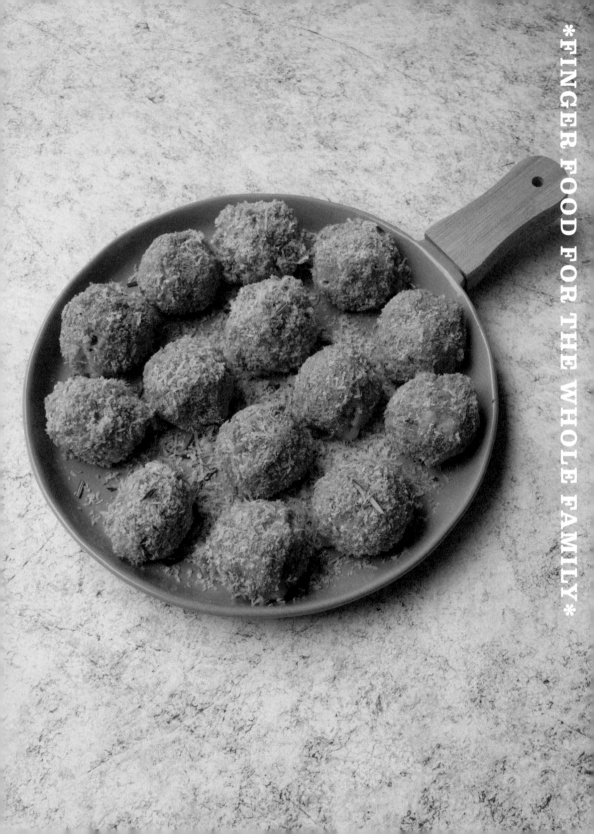

Asparagus, Spinach, Spring Onion and Pea Frittata

This frittata is packed full of greens and is a great option for baby and adult alike. Cut into little fingers when it's out of the oven for the perfect on-the-move finger food.

MAKES ABOUT 12 PORTIONS
Prep time 10 minutes
Cook time: 20 minutes

* BATCH COOK ME!
* VEGETARIAN
* FAMILY-FRIENDLY

Ingredients

1 teaspoon olive oil

3–4 spring onions/scallions, thinly sliced

3–4 asparagus spears, woody ends removed, thinly sliced

1 teaspoon dried or fresh oregano

1 teaspoon dried or fresh basil

Large handful of spinach leaves, finely chopped

100g/3½oz/½ cup frozen peas

5 large eggs, beaten

100g/3½oz/¾ cup Cheddar cheese, grated

2 tablespoons plain/all-purpose white flour (or any alternative)

1 Preheat the oven to 180°C/350°F/ Gas 4. Line a baking pan with non-stick baking paper.

2 Heat the oil in a pan over a medium heat. Add the spring onions/scallions and asparagus and fry for a few minutes. Add the oregano and basil, spinach and peas and cook for a further 2 minutes.

3 In a bowl, combine the eggs and Cheddar along with the flour, then mix in the cooked vegetables.

4 Pour the mixture into the lined baking pan and bake in the oven for around 15 mins until firm. Remove and leave to cool before cutting into slices.

>> **MIX IT UP:**
* Almost any vegetable works well here. Try some diced sweet potato, kale, peppers, courgette/ zucchini and sweetcorn.
* For an adult version add some green chillies or hot sauce.

Banana, Blueberry and Peanut Butter Loaf

There's nothing quite like the smell of banana bread baking in the house. This baby-friendly recipe includes blueberries, Greek yogurt and peanut butter and contains absolutely no added sugar. A delicious snack for both parents and baby to get stuck into.

MAKES 1 LOAF
Prep time: 10 minutes
Cook time: 50 minutes

* BATCH COOK ME!
* VEGETARIAN
* FAMILY-FRIENDLY

Ingredients

3 bananas
100g/3 ½oz Greek yogurt (or a
    plant-based alternative)
50ml/2fl oz/scant ¼ cup olive oil
1 egg, beaten
1 teaspoon ground cinnamon
100g/3½oz/1 cup blueberries
75g/2½oz/⅓ cup peanut butter
300g/10½oz/2 cups wholemeal/
    whole-wheat flour
2 teaspoons baking powder

1 Preheat the oven to 180°C/350°F/Gas 4 and grease a 900g/2lb loaf pan.

2 Mash the bananas together in a bowl and then add the yogurt, oil, egg, cinnamon and blueberries. Mix well.

3 Add the peanut butter and mix again. Sift in the flour and baking powder, mix once more, then spoon the mixture into the loaf pan.

4 Bake for around 50 minutes, then remove and leave to cool.

>> **MIX IT UP:**
* Almond butter works well instead of peanut butter.
* Swap the olive oil for coconut oil.
* Add some chopped dates, raisins and nuts for babies over one year old.

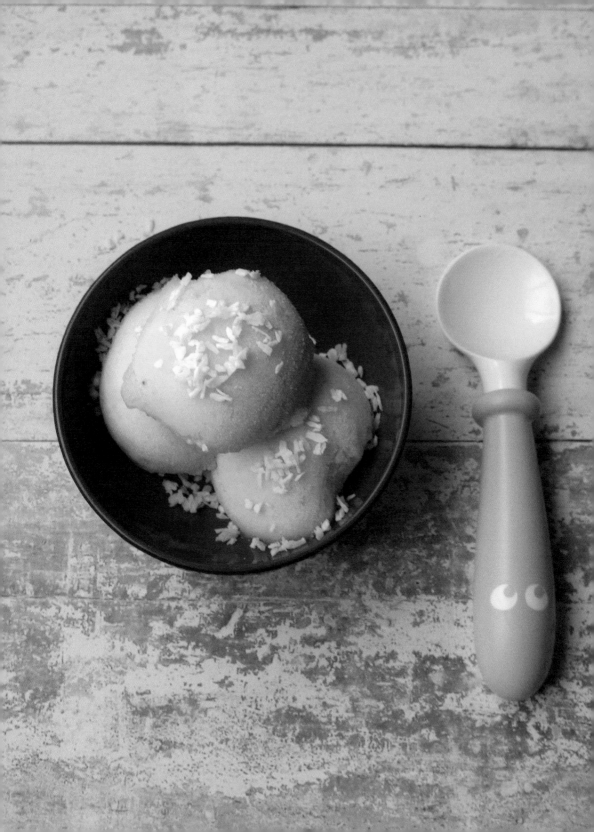

Banana and Mango "Ice Cream"

You may have noticed that there aren't many desserts around when it comes to feeding a baby. While anything with added sugar is off the cards, desserts are a great way to expose baby to different textures, temperatures and flavours. This dessert is made from frozen banana and mango, which when blended make a delicious ice cream alternative. Go slow and enjoy the look on your baby's face when they try something this cold for the first time!

MAKES 400ML /14FL OZ
Freezing time: 4 hours
Prep time: 5 minutes

✳ FAMILY-FRIENDLY

Ingredients
4 ripe bananas, sliced
1 mango, diced
1 teaspoon desiccated coconut

1 Place the bananas and mango in a freezer bag and freeze for at least 2 hours.

2 Transfer the fruit to a food processor and blend until creamy.

3 Freeze for another 2 hours in an airtight freezerproof container with a lid, then serve with a teaspoon of desiccated coconut on top. This will last in an airtight container in the freezer for 5–7 days.

>> **MIX IT UP:**
✳ Keep the banana as the base and play around with different fruits (but still chop them; a frozen whole strawberry will kill your food processor).
✳ Add a spoonful of nut butter when serving to add texture and nutrients.

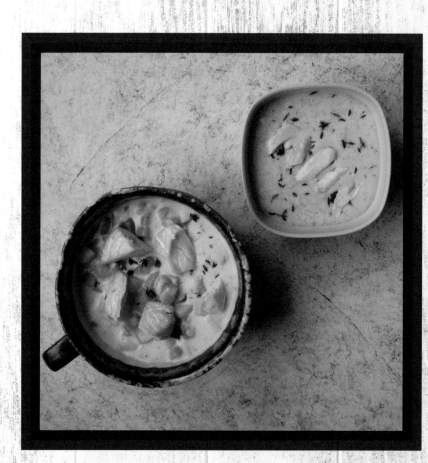

CHAPTER 6:
Meals for the
Whole Family
(8 months onwards)

Making Family Meals Baby-Friendly

With very few exceptions, all family meals can be easily adapted to become baby-friendly, and after a month or so of steaming vegetables non-stop this may be just what you want to do. Feeding baby the same food as the rest of the family not only encourages baby to try different foods (as everyone else is doing the same) but also cuts down on your cooking time enormously. Parents in the house may well be back at work, there may be other children to feed or, quite simply, there's just no desire to be stuck in the kitchen endlessly creating different meals for everyone. From 8 months onwards your baby can eat and digest pretty much any well-cooked food (see page 150 for any exceptions), so it's a great time to expose them to what the rest of the family is eating. If you have older children it's an ideal time to get them involved with helping their younger sibling to eat too.

What does baby need to eat?

A healthy diet for baby is pretty much the same as that of an adult, with a few exceptions. So as long as you are making healthy, balanced dishes for your family, then whatever you make will be suitable for your baby. Like adults, baby needs lots of vegetables, fruit, pulses/legumes, grains, meat, fish and dairy (unless you've chosen for baby to follow a plant-based diet). All of the main vitamins, protein, iron and omega-3 are crucially important to help them grow and develop, so have a look through previous chapter introductions if you need a refresher on which foods contain what.

Babies also need a lot of calcium to help build bones and keep teeth healthy, and fat for energy. As well as the recommended daily intake of milk, ensure your baby is eating lots of unsaturated fats (fish, blended nuts, seeds, avocado) yogurt and cheese – and always give your baby the full-fat option rather than a reduced- or low-fat product.

One dish for the whole family

You know best when it comes to what texture of food your baby can eat. Take a few spoonfuls of whatever dish you're making out of the pan when it's cooked and either blend to a purée, roughly mash with a fork or just allow it to cool. If you are following the baby-led-weaning approach, then put the bowl in front of baby and let them tuck in, obviously ensuring that there are no choking hazards in the dish. From around 9 months to a year, baby will be able to start using a spoon or fork themselves – although you'll obviously still need to help and they'll still make an absolute mess! If you're following a purée-led approach, then blend the dish to the right consistency and help them eat the dish with a spoon. Always serve some finger food alongside if you can, even if it's just spaghetti!

If you want to add salt to your food, always do so after you've taken a portion out for baby (although cooking for a baby is a great way to reduce your own salt intake). Avoid cooking with alcohol and while you should be exposing baby to different herbs and spices, don't give them anything spicy. If you want to eat anything that has added sugar or is heavily processed, then don't give it to baby.

Family-friendly recipes in this book

As well as the family-friendly meals listed in this chapter, many of the recipes that appear earlier in the book are perfectly suitable for baby to eat. Those that are have been clearly labelled as such. If you are cooking these dishes for baby, then remember to leave out the salt, or add it into the adult portions at the end, and to use a low-salt, baby-friendly stock if required.

SPOTLIGHT:

Weekend Breakfast Ideas

I initially called this section Weekend Brunch Ideas before remembering that both my children regularly wake up before 6am and by the time it's 10am, I'm already thinking about lunch. So, Weekend Breakfast Ideas it is!

I always like to make something a little different for breakfast over the weekend. There's no rush to get to nursery or work and we can all take a bit more time and enjoy eating together. It's also a good opportunity to take a break from porridge and I found that my sons really appreciated the change. In our house now we only make porridge when they're off to nursery; otherwise we have either cereal, nut butter on toast or a selection of the below. I hope you find these useful too.

French Toast with Raspberries and Mango

SERVES 3−4
Prep time: 10 minutes
Cook time: 15 minutes

* FAMILY-FRIENDLY

Ingredients
6 eggs * 1 tablespoon butter (or a plant-based alternative) * 1 loaf of brioche, sliced * 100–150g/3½–5½oz /1–1½ cups fresh raspberries, chopped * 1 mango, sliced

1 Beat the eggs in a wide bowl. Melt the butter in a frying pan over a medium heat. Dip one slice of brioche in the egg, press down, then flip and repeat. Place in the heated pan and cook for 2−3 minutes per side. Repeat with the rest of the brioche slices, cooking them in batches.

2 Once cooked, remove the French toast from the pan and top with the raspberries and mango.

3 Cut the french toast into fingers for baby.

Baby-Friendly Scrambled Eggs

SERVES 2–3
Prep time: 5 minutes
Cooking time: 7 minutes

✳ FAMILY-FRIENDLY

Ingredients

1 teaspoon butter (or a plant-based alternative)
✳ 1 shallot, finely chopped ✳ 1 garlic clove,
finely chopped ✳ 1–2 tomatoes, finely chopped
✳ 1 teaspoon chopped oregano ✳ 5 eggs ✳
30–50g/1–1¾oz/¼–⅓ cup Cheddar cheese
grated ✳ A few slices of wholegrain bread

1 Melt the butter in a pan over a medium heat. Add the shallot, garlic, tomatoes and oregano and cook for a couple of minutes.

2 Beat the eggs in a bowl. Add the cooked tomato mixture, stir well, then pour back into the pan.

3 Cook the eggs over a medium heat for a few minutes then remove from the heat and leave in the pan for 2–3 minutes until they're cooked through.

4 Add the grated Cheddar to the eggs and mix well. Serve with some wholegrain bread.

Banana and Blueberry Pancakes with Cinnamon Bananas and Yogurt

MAKES ABOUT 12 PANCAKES
Prep time: 10 minutes
Cook time: 20 minutes per pancake

✳ BATCH COOK ME!
✳ FAMILY-FRIENDLY

Ingredients

30g/1¾oz butter (or a plant-based alternative),
plus 2 teaspoons for cooking ✳ 3 eggs
✳ 400ml/14fl oz/1 ⅔ cups full-fat/whole milk
(or a plant-based alternative) ✳ 3 bananas
✳ 50g/1¾oz/⅓ cup rolled oats ✳ 200g/7oz/
2 cups fresh blueberries, plus extra for topping
✳ 200g/7oz/1⅓ cups wholemeal/whole-wheat
flour (or any gluten-free alternative) ✳ 3 teaspoons
baking powder ✳ 1 teaspoon ground cinnamon

✳ Greek yogurt, for topping (or a plant-based alternative) ✳ Maple syrup, for topping (for those over one year old only)

Please note:
Any uncooked blueberries served to baby should be quartered. Maple syrup is not recommended for children under one year old.

1 Melt the butter, ensure it's cooled, then pour into a bowl and whisk together with the eggs and milk.

2 Mash 2 of the bananas with a fork

and add to the bowl along with the oats.

3 Melt a teaspoon of butter in a frying pan over a high heat. Add the blueberries and cook for 2 minutes until they go all squishy and are now suitable for baby to eat whole. Add them to the bowl.

4 Sift the flour and baking powder into the bowl and stir a few times until you have a batter.

5 Melt another teaspoon of butter in the pan, then add a ladleful of the batter. Cook for around 3 minutes until air bubbles appear on the top of the pancake, then flip it over and cook for another 2 minutes. Repeat with the rest of the batter, cooking the pancakes in batches. Add more butter to the pan between batches if you need to.

6 Slice the remaining banana and sprinkle the cinnamon over the top. Serve the pancakes with Greek yogurt, the sliced bananas, fresh blueberries and maple syrup (for those over one year old).

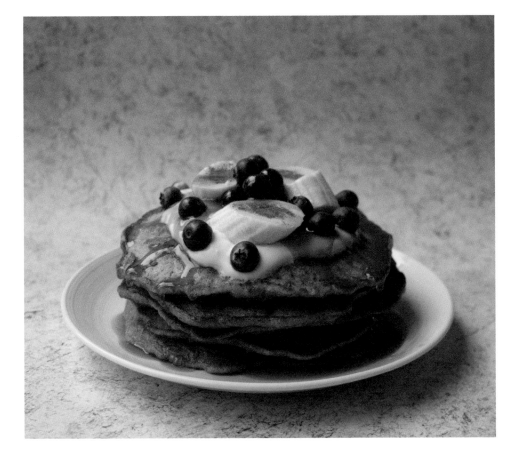

>> **MIX IT UP:**

* If your little one is wolfing down chicken easily, cut it into cubes.

* For a vegetarian option, roast the broccoli, then cut into very small pieces and stir through.

Pea, Broccoli and Shredded Lemon Chicken Risotto

Young tums sometimes find it hard to digest big chunks of protein, so to get around this I started shredding chicken and stirring it through dishes. It works well for when baby has begun to eat the same meal as you. I also set aside a few strips of chicken for finger food. See page 178 for how to make arancini from leftover risotto.

SERVES 2 adults plus lots of portions for baby, the rest of the family or the freezer

Prep time: 10 minutes

Cook time: 30 minutes

✱ BATCH COOK ME!

✱ FAMILY-FRIENDLY

Ingredients

4 chicken breasts

Juice of 1 lemon

1 tablespoon olive oil

1 onion, diced

2 garlic cloves, crushed

1 teaspoon fresh or dried chopped sage

A knob of butter

250g/9oz/1 cup Arborio rice

800ml/28fl oz/scant 3½ cups baby-friendly chicken stock

75g/2½oz/½ cup broccoli florets

150g/5½oz/¾ cups frozen peas

A few tablespoons of Parmesan cheese, grated

1 Preheat the oven to 180°C/350°F/Gas 4.

2 Place the chicken breasts on a baking sheet and squeeze over the lemon juice. (You shouldn't use salt in a dish for a baby, so lemon adds flavour and also stops the chicken drying out.) Bake for 25 minutes, turning halfway, then remove and leave to cool slightly. Slice a few chicken strips for finger food. Shred the rest with two forks and set aside.

3 Meanwhile, heat the oil in a pan over a medium heat. Add the onion and cook for 2–3 minutes. Add the garlic, sage and butter, mix well, then add the rice, mix well again and cook for 2 minutes.

4 Add a ladleful of stock and stir well until most has been absorbed, then add another ladleful and repeat until all the stock has been used up (this will take about 20 minutes).

5 Meanwhile, cook the broccoli in a separate pan of boiling water for 3–4 minutes. Drain, then chop and add to the risotto.

6 Put the peas in a bowl. Pour over hot water to defrost them. Add half to the risotto. Blend, or mash with a fork, the rest and set aside.

7 When the risotto is cooked, remove from the heat. Stir in the remaining peas and shredded chicken. Top with Parmesan. Season the adult portions as required.

Sausage, Butter Bean and Kale Hotpot

Sausages are a real weekend food in our house, and this is a dish I make regularly. Loads of veg, a nice, warming broth and the start of a life-long love affair with sausages.

SERVES 2, plus a few baby portions

Prep time: 15 minutes
Cook time: 35 minutes

✳ BATCH COOK ME!
✳ FAMILY-FRIENDLY

Ingredients

2 tablespoons olive oil
8 good-quality butchers' sausages (pork or vegan)
1 shallot, diced
1 teaspoon thyme
1 teaspoon rosemary
1 teaspoon oregano
2 courgettes/zucchini, finely diced
2 carrots, finely diced
1 tablespoon plain/all-purpose white flour (or any alternative)
600ml/20fl oz/2½ cups vegetable stock
2 large handfuls of kale, tough stalks removed, roughly chopped
2 x 400g/14oz can of butter/lima beans, drained
Crusty bread, to serve

1 Heat 1 tablespoon of the oil in a large frying pan over a medium heat. Add the sausages and cook for around 5–6 minutes, turning once. Remove, then wipe away any excess fat from the pan.

2 Heat the remaining tablespoon of the oil in the pan. Add the shallot and cook for 2–3 minutes. Add the thyme, rosemary and oregano and mix well. Add the courgettes/zucchini and carrots and cook for 3–4 minutes.

3 Whisk the flour into the stock, then pour into the pan. Add the sausages back in, cover the pan and simmer for 15 minutes.

4 Add the kale and butter/lima beans and cook for a further 3–4 minutes.

5 Serve with some crusty bread. For baby, whizz up a few spoonfuls of the vegetables along with half a sausage for a delicious purée.

>> **MIX IT UP:**
✳ Swap the sausages for some thickly cut chunks of pork, or use vegetarian sausages for a veggie option.
✳ Serve over brown rice or add in some pasta shells for extra carbs.
✳ Grate some cheese into the dish. Swap the butter/lima beans for cannellini or borlotti beans.

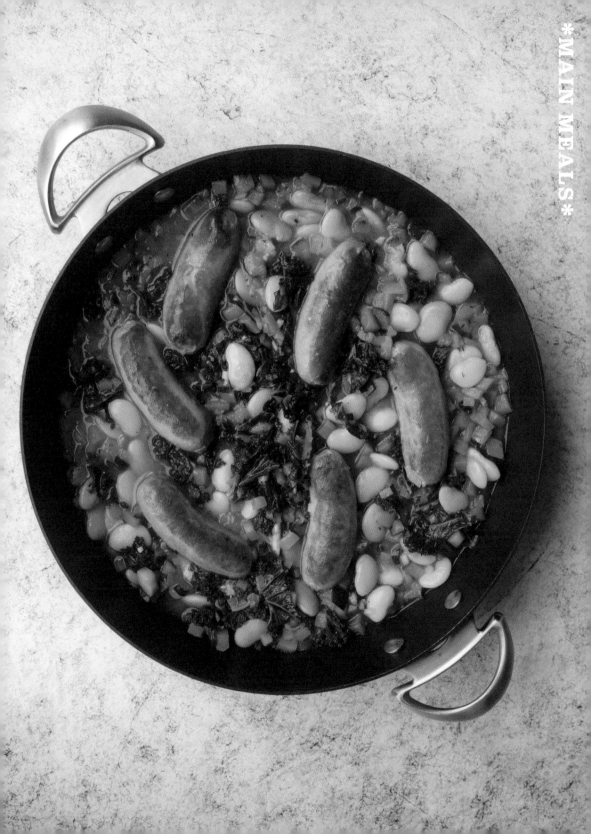

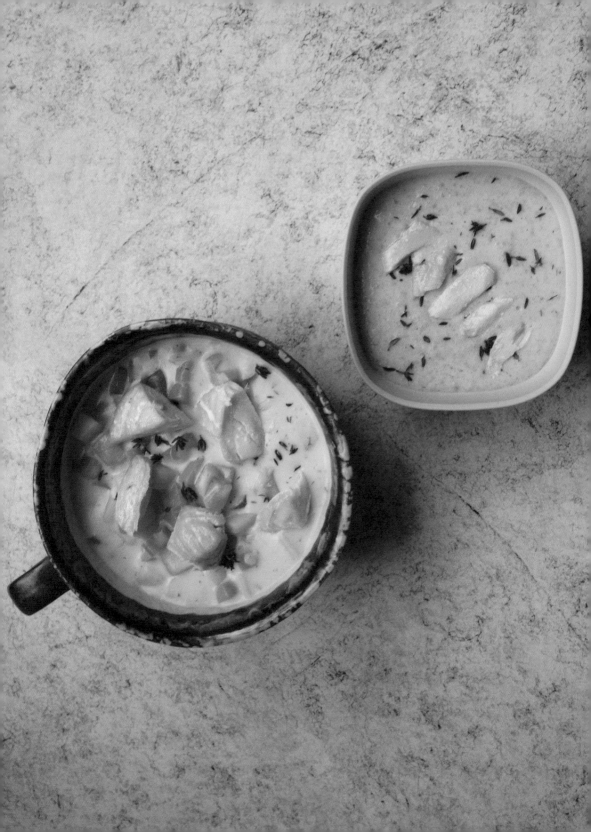

Salmon Chowder

A warming bowl of comfort food right here, and a delicious family meal. This is a really enjoyable dish to make and one that's full of nutrients for baby. It's a great introduction to different herbs and textures – plus seeing them nibble on some salmon as finger food makes your heart burst with joy!

SERVES 2, plus a few baby portions
Prep time: 10 minutes
Cook time: 20 minutes

✳ FAMILY-FRIENDLY

Ingredients
A knob of butter
1 shallot, diced
1 teaspoon dried thyme
1 teaspoon dried sage
2 large potatoes, peeled and cut into 1cm/½in dice
2 carrots, finely diced
4 celery stalks, finely diced
200ml/7fl oz/scant 1 cup vegetable stock
3 salmon fillets, about 150g/5½oz each
Juice of ½ lemon
1 tablespoon plain/all-purpose white flour (or any alternative)
400ml/10½fl oz/1¼ cups full-fat/whole milk (or any plant-based alternative)
50g/1¾oz/⅓ cup Cheddar cheese

1 Preheat the oven to 180°C/350°F/Gas 4.

2 Melt the butter in a saucepan over a medium heat. Add the shallot and cook for 2–3 minutes. Add the thyme and sage and mix well.

3 Add the potatoes, carrots and celery, then pour over the vegetable stock and cook for 10 minutes until the vegetables are nice and soft.

4 Meanwhile, place the salmon fillets on a baking sheet and squeeze over a little lemon juice. Bake for 10 minutes, then remove and flake into small pieces.

5 Whisk the flour into the milk, then pour into the pan. Cook for another 5 minutes. Divide between 2 bowls and top with the salmon. For baby, blend a spoonful or two of the chowder to your preferred consistency and top with some flaked salmon to use as finger food.

> > **MIX IT UP:**
> ✳ Swap the potatoes for celeriac or cauliflower.
> ✳ Add some sweetcorn.
> ✳ A vegetarian option is to use a dozen or so asparagus stalks instead of salmon.

Mackerel Kedgeree

Mackerel is a great fish for baby to eat, as it's packed full of protein, omega-3 and lots of other nutrients. There's a little spice here but nothing to blow baby's socks off, plus it's fun to watch them try to pick up half a runny soft-boiled egg!

SERVES 2, plus a few
baby-sized portions
Prep time: 10 minutes
Cook time: 25 minutes

* BATCH COOK ME!
* FAMILY-FRIENDLY

Ingredients

A knob of butter

1 leek, thinly sliced

1 teaspoon mustard seeds

1 teaspoon ground turmeric

1 teaspoon garam masala

1 teaspoon ground cumin

1 teaspoon ground coriander

200g/7oz/generous 1 cup brown
basmati rice

500ml/17fl oz/2 cups
vegetable stock

100g/3½oz/½ cup frozen peas

4 eggs

2 smoked mackerel fillets, about
180g each, skin removed

A few chives, chopped

A few coriander/cilantro sprigs,
leaves chopped

1 Melt the butter in a pan over a low heat. Add the leek and cook for 5 minutes. Stir in the spices and cook for another minute or so. Add the rice and stir well.

2 Add the stock to the pan, cover and cook for about 20 minutes, adding more water if the pan runs dry. Add the peas to the pan after 15 minutes of cooking. Just before you've finished cooking the kedgeree, flake the mackerel and mix it in gently to warm through.

3 Meanwhile, cook the eggs to your preference. I like them soft-boiled, so I cook them for around 6 minutes in boiling water, then drain and leave in a bowl of iced water until needed.

4 Remove the pan from the heat. Peel the eggs, cut into quarters and place on top. Sprinkle over the chives and coriander/cilantro. For baby, mash the rice with a fork to your desired consistency and use some of the mackerel as finger food. If freezing, don't include the eggs.

> > **MIX IT UP:**
> * Swap in some cooked salmon instead of the mackerel, if you prefer.
> * Add some more diced vegetables to the kedgeree, such as carrots or celery.
> * Serve with some fresh yogurt and, if cooking for adults only, add a green chilli at the end for a bit more heat.

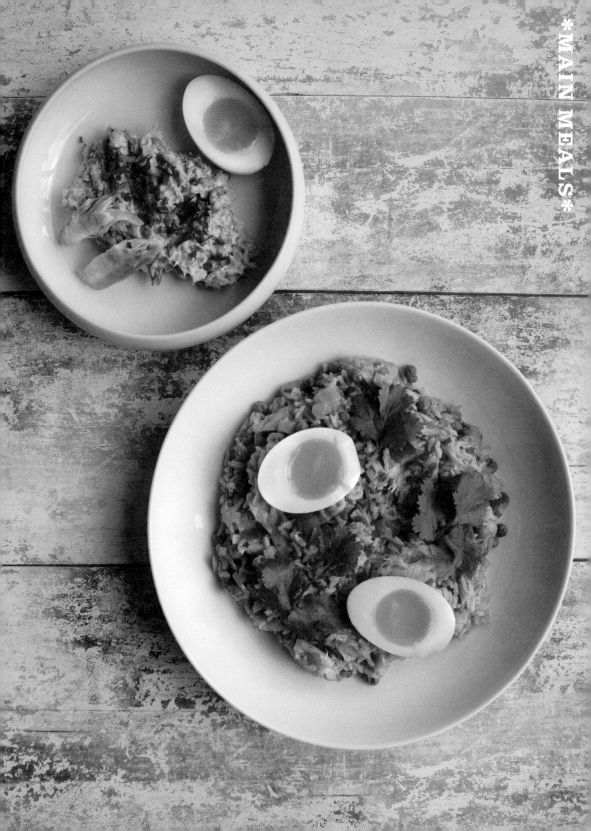

>> **MIX IT UP:**
* Any vegetables work here: frozen sweetcorn, grated carrot, celery or whatever is in your vegetable drawer.

Italian Chicken and Vegetable Pasta Bake

A very easy one-pot dish. Baby will love playing with the large rigatoni pasta, which because of the melted cheese will have lots of vegetables stuck to it. If everything is cut small enough, just place a bowl in front of baby and let them experiment while you dig into yours.

MAKES 2–3 adult-sized portions, plus a few baby-sized portions too
Prep time: 15 minutes
Cook time: 50 minutes

✱ BATCH COOK ME!
✱ FAMILY-FRIENDLY

Ingredients

2 tablespoons olive oil
8 chicken thighs, preferably de-boned
Juice of 1 lemon
500g/1lb 2oz whole-wheat rigatoni
    (or penne or fusilli would work well)
1 onion, diced
2 garlic cloves, finely chopped
12 pitted green olives, finely chopped
1 teaspoon oregano
2 red peppers, cored, deseeded and
    finely diced
1 courgette/zucchini, finely diced
6–8 chestnut/cremini mushrooms,
    finely diced
2 x 400g/14oz canned tomatoes
1 tablespoon tomato purée/paste
70g/2½ oz/½ cup Parmesan cheese,
    grated
100g/3½oz/½ cup frozen peas
250g/9oz mozzarella
100g/3½oz/1 cup Panko
    breadcrumbs
A few parsley sprigs, leaves chopped

1 Preheat the oven to 180°C/350°F/Gas 4.

2 Heat a tablespoon of the oil in a frying pan over a medium heat. Add the chicken thighs, squeeze over the lemon juice and cook for around 15–18 minutes, turning once, until cooked through. Set aside. Once cool, use two forks to shred the chicken into small pieces, removing the bone if necessary.

3 Meanwhile, cook the pasta for 2 minutes less than the packet instructions, then drain and set aside.

4 Heat the remaining oil in the pan over a medium heat. Add the onion and cook for 2–3 minutes. Add the garlic, olives, oregano, peppers, courgette/zucchini and mushrooms and cook for 5 minutes.

5 Stir in the canned tomatoes and tomato purée/paste, then cover and cook for 20 minutes.

6 Stir in half the Parmesan, the peas, shredded chicken and cooked pasta. Mix everything together well.

7 Pour the pasta mix into a large ovenproof dish and tear or grate over the mozzarella. Sprinkle with the remaining Parmesan and breadcrumbs. Cook for 20 minutes.

8 Serve sprinkled with parsley on top.

Lentil, Mushroom and Kale Lasagne

Lasagne is such a versatile dish and a great way of getting lots of veg into baby. Pasta sheets make excellent finger food and the dish is hearty enough to give tired parents an energy boost too!

SERVES 2, plus a few baby portions and some for the freezer
Prep time: 15 minutes
Cook time: 50 minutes

✳ BATCH COOK ME!
✳ VEGETARIAN
✳ FAMILY-FRIENDLY

Ingredients

1 teaspoon olive oil
1 shallot, diced
2 garlic cloves, finely chopped
1 tablespoon oregano, fresh or dried
500g/1lb 2oz/7½ cups chestnut/cremini mushrooms, trimmed and finely diced
2 x 400g/14oz cans chopped tomatoes
1 tablespoon tomato purée/paste
250g/9oz kale, tough stalks removed, roughly chopped
2 x 400g/14oz cans green lentils, drained
50g/1¾ oz/scant ¼ cup butter (or plant-based alternative)
50g/1¾oz/⅓ cup plain/all-purpose white flour (or any alternative)
400ml/14fl oz/1 ⅔ cups full-fat/whole milk (or a plant-based alternative)
200g/7oz/1½ cups Cheddar, grated
Enough lasagne sheets for 2 layers in your dish, wholegrain if you can
150g/5½oz /1 ½ cups mozzarella

1 Preheat the oven to 180°C/350°F/Gas 4.

2 Heat the oil in a frying pan over a low heat. Add the shallot and cook for a couple of minutes. Add the garlic, oregano and mushrooms. Cook for 2–3 minutes. Add the tomatoes and tomato purée/paste and cook for 7–8 minutes. Add the kale and lentils.

3 Make your bechamel sauce. Melt the butter in a saucepan over a medium heat. Add the flour and let it cook for a minute or so until the pan begins to smell like a cookie! Little by little, pour the milk into the pan, taking it on and off the heat and whisking continuously. When you've used up all the milk, let the sauce cook for a further 2 minutes before removing from the heat. Add the Cheddar and mix well.

4 Spoon half of the mushroom and kale mixture into the bottom of an ovenproof dish. Cover with a layer of lasagne sheets, then pour over half of the bechamel. Spoon the rest of the mushroom and kale mixture on top, followed by another layer of lasagne sheets and then the remaining bechamel. Top with the grated mozzarella and bake for 30 minutes.

>> **MIX IT UP:**
∗ Add more veg to the lasagne, such as diced courgettes/zucchini, peppers and carrots or swap the kale for spinach.
∗ Of course, minced/ground beef or lamb works well too.

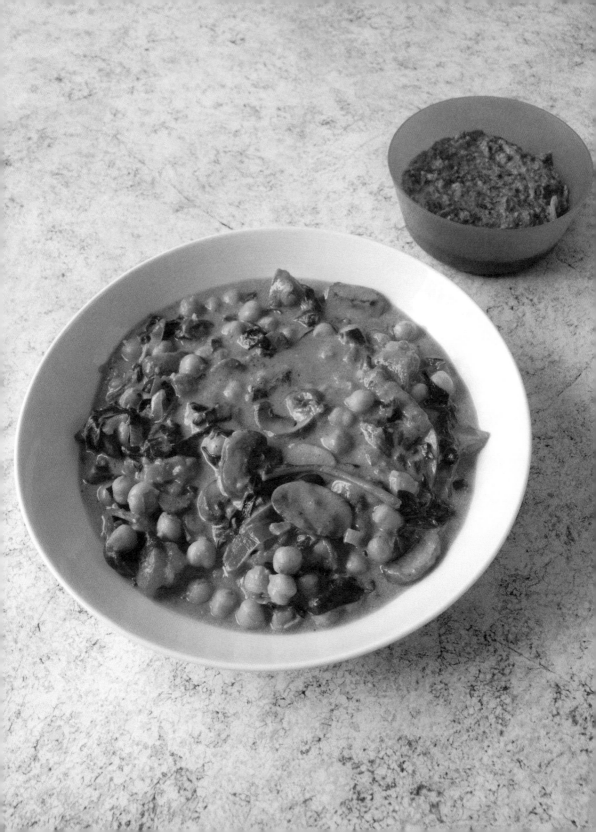

Mushroom, Chickpea and Spinach Curry

This is a really fun, nutritious and easy-to-make dish suitable for the whole family. It's a great, plant-based way to introduce some gentle spices to baby. Making mushrooms the star of the dish means that everyone is getting a dose of vitamin D too. Serve over rice if you like.

SERVES 2, plus a few baby portions

Prep time: 10 minutes

Cook time: 20 minutes

* BATCH COOK ME!
* VEGAN/VEGETARIAN
* FAMILY-FRIENDLY

Ingredients

1 tablespoon vegetable oil

1 shallot, diced

5cm/2in piece of fresh root ginger, peeled and finely grated

2 garlic cloves, crushed

1 teaspoon ground turmeric

1 teaspoon garam masala

1 teaspoon ground coriander

1 teaspoon ground cumin

1 teaspoon mustard seeds

12 chestnut/cremini mushrooms, thinly sliced

1 x 400ml/14fl oz can of coconut milk

2 tomatoes, sliced

2 x 400g/14oz cans of chickpeas/ garbanzo beans, drained

2 large handfuls of spinach leaves, chopped

1 Heat the oil in a frying pan over a low heat. Add the shallot and fry for a couple of minutes. Add the ginger, garlic, turmeric, garam masala, ground coriander, cumin and mustard seeds. Stir well so the spices coat the shallot.

2 Add the mushrooms and cook for another 2 minutes. Add the coconut milk and cook for 8–10 minutes so it starts to reduce. Add the tomatoes and cook for a further 2 minutes. Finally, add the chickpeas/garbanzo beans and the spinach and cook for 2 more minutes before serving.

>> **MIX IT UP:**
* Add tofu or, for a non-vegan option, add some paneer to the pan when cooking. Tofu and paneer make great finger foods too.

Quesadillas!

Quesadillas are for the whole family to enjoy! They're really versatile, super quick to make if you have some leftover fillings to use up and are a brilliant finger food for your baby. Make sure to cook them for a good 3–4 minutes on each side so it's easier for baby to hold. The classic quesadilla contains just melted cheese and mashed avocado, but you can really put anything in them. Here, I've added some spiced shredded chicken, smashed sweetcorn, avocado, mozzarella and coriander/cilantro but this is also a great way of using up leftovers.

SERVES 2, plus a few portions
for baby
Prep time: 15 minutes
Cook time: 40 minutes

✳ FAMILY-FRIENDLY

Ingredients

1 teaspoon ground cumin
1 teaspoon smoked paprika
1 teaspoon oregano
2 chicken breasts
100g/3½oz/½ cup frozen sweetcorn
2 avocados, peeled and destoned
6 wholemeal/whole-wheat tortillas
250g/9oz /2½ cups mozzarella,
grated or thinly sliced
A few coriander/cilantro sprigs,
leaves finely chopped

1 Heat the oven to 180°C/350°F/Gas 4. Mix the chicken, cumin, paprika and oregano together in a bowl then tip onto a baking tray and cook in the oven for 15 minutes until piping hot throughout. Remove, leave to cool, and then shred.

2 Place the frozen sweetcorn in a bowl and cover with boiling water. Leave for 3–4 minutes, then drain and mash with a fork. In a separate bowl, mash the avocados.

3 Lay one of the tortillas on a flat surface. Spread half of the tortilla with avocado and top with some of the sweetcorn, chicken and mozzarella. Fold over the other half of the tortilla and press down. In a hot frying pan over a medium heat, dry-fry the quesadilla for 3–4 minutes on each side. Always cook quesadillas cheese-side down first.

4 Use a pizza cutter to cut the quesadillas into finger-sized portions for baby and cover with some chopped coriander/cilantro.

>> **MIX IT UP:**

* Anything goes here, just make sure it's cut into small enough pieces so it doesn't become a choking hazard. How about:
* Add diced onions and peppers to the chicken mix.
* Cook some black beans, butter/lima beans, kidney beans or chickpeas/garbanzo beans in the same mix, then mash well.
* Pulled pork or diced prawns/shrimp instead of the chicken, or some roasted squash or pumpkin for a veggie option.

Sausage and Vegetable Carbonara

This is a perfect Sunday evening dish to round off the weekend and set you all up for the week ahead. Babies will love the creamy carbonara, and if you use penne, it's perfect for them to pick up — hopefully along with some lovely diced veg stuck on!

SERVES 2, plus lots of
portions for baby
Prep time: 10 minutes
Cook time: 20 minutes

✳ BATCH COOK ME!
✳ FAMILY-FRIENDLY

Ingredients

2 tablespoons olive oil
8 good-quality butchers' sausages
(pork or vegan)
300g/10½oz pasta (penne, rigatoni,
casarecce or a similar-sized pasta)
1 shallot, diced
2 garlic cloves, finely chopped
1 teaspoon chopped rosemary
6–8 chestnut mushrooms, finely diced
1 yellow pepper, cored, deseeded
and finely diced
100g/3½oz/½ cup frozen peas
2 egg yolks
40g/1½oz/⅓ cup Parmesan, grated
5 tablespoons full-fat/whole milk (or a
plant-based alternative)
A few parsley sprigs, leaves chopped

> > **MIX IT UP:**
✳ Use finely chopped
vegetables (broccoli,
spinach, etc) instead of
sausage for a veggie option;
just make sure to cook hard
veg like carrot thoroughly.

1 Heat a tablespoon of the oil in a frying pan over a medium heat. Add the sausages and fry for around 8–10 minutes, turning a few times. Place the sausages on some paper towels and wipe away any excess fat from the pan.

2 Meanwhile, cook the pasta as per the packet instructions, then drain, reserving a few tablespoons of the cooking water, and set aside.

3 Heat a tablespoon of oil in the pan over a low heat. Add the shallot and cook for a few minutes. Add the garlic and the rosemary and cook for a minute. Add the mushrooms, pepper and peas and cook for 5 minutes.

4 Slice the sausages, then add to the pan along with 2–3 tablespoons of the pasta cooking water. Cook for a further 2–3 minutes to ensure the sausages are cooked completely.

5 Using a fork in a bowl, beat the eggs yolks together with the Parmesan and the milk.

6 Add the cooked pasta to the pan. Pour over the carbonara sauce, toss everything together well, cook for a further minute, then remove the pan from the heat and let it stand for a few minutes. The heat of the pan will fully cook the egg yolks. Sprinkle over the parsley.

7 Make either a purée for baby or place a few spoonfuls in a bowl for baby-led-weaning. If baby is feeding themselves, make sure you finely chop the sausages before serving.

Chicken Schnitzel with Best-Ever Potato Wedges and Marinara Dip

A weekend dish for the whole family! The wedges are to die for, and the marinara sauce is full of good stuff. Baby can easily hold, play with and eat the breaded chicken strips and potato wedges.

SERVES 2, plus a few baby or child-sized portions

Prep time: 15 minutes

Cook time: 45 minutes

* BATCH COOK ME!
* FAMILY-FRIENDLY

Ingredients

5–6 large white potatoes, peeled

2 tablespoons olive oil

100g/3½oz/¾ cup Parmesan, grated

2 tablespoons dried oregano

4 garlic cloves, finely chopped

1 onion, diced

1 x 400g/14oz can chopped tomatoes

2–3 tablespoons chopped thyme

3 chicken breasts

2 eggs

100g/3½oz/⅔ cup plain/all-purpose white flour (or any alternative)

100g/3½oz/1 cup panko breadcrumbs

2 tablespoons vegetable oil

A handful of parsley, chopped

1 Preheat the oven to 200°C/400°F/Gas 6. Line 2 large baking trays with baking paper.

2 Slice the potatoes in half width-ways, then cut each piece in half. Cut each piece in half again so you have 8 equal wedges per potato. Mix in a bowl along with the oil, ⅔ of the Parmesan, half of the oregano and half of the garlic. Lay the wedges out on the baking trays and roast for 35 minutes, turning once.

3 To make the marinara dip, fry the onion in the remaining oil for 3 minutes. Add the remaining garlic and oregano, stir, then add the tomatoes. Cook for 20 minutes to reduce then serve as it is or blend for a smooth dip.

4 Meanwhile, slice each chicken breast in half width-ways so you have 6 thin chicken portions. Then cut each into 3 or 4 pieces.

5 In a wide bowl, whisk the eggs. Place the flour and breadcrumbs in two separate bowls. Dip each piece of chicken in the flour, then the egg and finally the breadcrumbs, ensuring it is completely covered. Heat a splash of vegetable oil in a pan and when hot, fry the chicken for around 8 minutes, turning once. Don't crowd the pan; you'll probably cook around 5–6 pieces per batch. Place the cooked chicken on kitchen paper while you cook the rest.

6 Sprinkle the cooked wedges with more Parmesan and parsley. Serve with the dip.

>> **MIX IT UP:**
* Swap the prawns/
shrimp for chicken or tofu.
* Swap the noodles for
wholegrain rice.

Family-Friendly Prawn Yaki Soba

Stir-fries are so easy to make and a treasure chest of excitement for babies exploring tastes and textures. However, most stir-fry marinades aren't baby-friendly because they tend to be high in salt, chilli, processed sugars or honey (remember, no honey until baby is over one). This recipe not only tastes good but is baby-friendly too.

SERVES 2, plus lots of baby
    portions
Prep time: 10 minutes
Cook time: 25 minutes

✳ BATCH COOK ME!
✳ FAMILY-FRIENDLY

Ingredients

200g/7oz whole-wheat noodles
2 garlic cloves, crushed
5cm/2in piece of fresh root
    ginger, peeled and grated
2 teaspoons low-salt soy sauce
3 teaspoons sesame oil
1 shallot, diced
1 large carrot, sliced into matchsticks
2 peppers, preferably different colours,
    cored, deseeded and finely sliced
    into matchsticks
4–6 mushrooms, trimmed and finely
    diced
100g/3½oz/½ cup frozen peas
100g/3½oz/½ cup frozen sweetcorn
250g/9oz raw peeled king prawns/
    jumbo shrimp
Juice of ½ lemon
A knob of butter (or plant-based
    alternative)
2 eggs, beaten
2 spring onions/scallions, thinly sliced
1 tablespoon sesame seeds

1 Prepare the noodles as per the packet instructions, then drain and set aside.

2 For the sauce, mix one of the garlic cloves and the ginger in a bowl. Add the soy sauce and 2 teaspoons of the oil, then set aside.

3 Heat the remaining teaspoon of oil in a frying pan over a medium heat. Add the shallot and cook for a couple of minutes. Add the garlic and carrot and cook for a few more minutes.

4 Add the peppers, mushrooms, peas and sweetcorn. Cook for 6–8 minutes.

5 Add the prawns/shrimp and the sauce. Squeeze over the lemon juice and cook for 5 minutes until the prawns are cooked through.

6 Meanwhile, in a separate pan, melt the butter and add the eggs. Move the pan around to spread the mixture out evenly and create a thin omelette. It should only take a few minutes to cook. Remove from the pan and cut into strips.

7 Add the noodles and the sliced omelette to the stir fry and mix everything together.

8 Sprinkle over the spring onions/scallions and sesame seeds before serving. Make either a purée for baby or place a few spoonfuls in a bowl for baby-led-weaning. They'll love pulling at the noodles, exploring the vegetables and nibbling on the prawns.

Cod, Orzo, Courgette and Tomato Traybake with Pistou

I've only got into orzo recently and I've found it to be really family-friendly. The dish makes great finger food for baby and the flavours also combine well in a purée. It's packed full of nutrients from the cod and vegetables, and the pistou adds a little zing to the dish.

SERVES 2–3, plus lots of baby portions

Prep time: 10 minutes

Cook time: 30 minutes

✳ FAMILY-FRIENDLY

Ingredients

100ml/3½fl oz/scant ½ cup olive oil

1 shallot, finely chopped

3 garlic cloves, crushed

1 teaspoon of dried oregano

2 courgettes/zucchini, diced

12 cherry tomatoes

600ml/21fl oz/2½ cups baby-friendly vegetable stock

300g/10½oz/1½ cups orzo

1 lemon, sliced

3–4 cod loins or fillets

Large handful of basil leaves

> **>> MIX IT UP:**
> ✳ Swap the pistou for your chosen pesto.
> ✳ Swap the cod for any other white fish or replace with roasted cauliflower, tofu or broccoli for a plant-based option.

1 Preheat the oven to 180°C/350°F/Gas 4.

2 Heat a teaspoon of the oil in a frying pan over a medium heat. Add the shallot and cook for 2–3 minutes before adding 1 clove of garlic and oregano. Mix well, then add the courgettes and tomatoes to the pan and cook for a further 3 minutes.

3 Add the orzo to the pan and mix well. Transfer to a deep ovenproof dish, then pour over the stock. Bake for around 20 minutes until the stock has been mostly absorbed. Top up with additional stock if the orzo runs dry before it's cooked.

4 Arrange the lemon slices on a baking sheet. Place the cod on top and roast in the oven for around 12 minutes.

5 Using a mini food processor blend the remaining garlic, basil and olive oil to make the pistou. Set aside.

6 Serve the cod on top of the orzo with some pistou drizzled over. Make either a purée for baby or place a few spoonfuls in a bowl for baby-led-weaning.

Banana, Blueberry and Oat Cookies

Who doesn't love a cookie? These have no added sugar and are packed full of fibre and nutrients. They are suitable for babies over 6 months and the rest of the family will love them too. Make loads and keep some in the freezer.

MAKES 12 COOKIES
Prep time: 5 minutes
Cook time: 20 minutes

✳ BATCH COOK ME!
✳ FAMILY-FRIENDLY

Ingredients
160g/5½oz/1½ cup rolled oats
2 bananas, mashed
100g/3½oz/1 cup blueberries
1 tablespoon chia seeds

1 Heat the oven to 180°C/350°F/Gas 4. Line a baking pan with non-stick baking paper.

2 In a bowl, mix together the oats, bananas, blueberries and chia seeds.

3 Shape the mixture into 12 golf-ball-sized balls with your hands. Place on the lined baking pan and press down on each ball slightly to create a cookie shape. Bake for 20 minutes.

>> **MIX IT UP:**
✳ If you're comfortable with your kids having chocolate (we waited until they were 1 year old then did it sparingly) add 60g of chocolate chips to the mixture.
✳ Grate in some courgette/zucchini or carrot.
✳ If your child is 1 year or older, you could add some seeds, dried fruit, raisins, grated citrus zest, cardamon or chopped nuts.

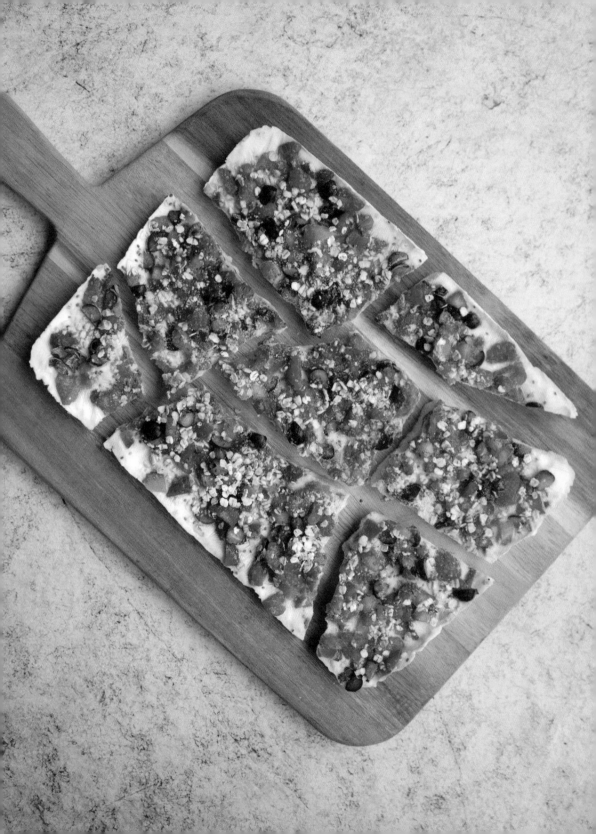

Frozen Yogurt, Mixed Berry and Oat Bark

This gets messy, but baby will have an absolute blast trying to nibble this yogurt bark. It's a great way to introduce different temperatures and textures. Make sure the berries are chopped small enough, to the size that you're comfortable with for your child (this is dependent on age). Make lots of little portions for the freezer, then remove a piece and let it soften slightly before giving to baby.

MAKES ENOUGH TO FILL ONE DISH of around 30cm/12in x 20cm/8in

Prep time: 10 minutes plus 4 hours freezing

✳ BATCH COOK ME!
✳ FAMILY-FRIENDLY

Ingredients

500g/1lb 2oz/2 cups Greek yogurt (or a plant-based alternative)
200g/7oz/1⅓ cups combination of raspberries, blueberries and strawberries, very finely chopped
30g/1oz/⅓ cup rolled oats
2 tablespoons chia seeds

1 Line a freezer-safe dish (around 30cm x 20cm/12in x 8in) with kitchen foil. Spoon the yogurt into the dish and spread out evenly. You're looking for a thickness of around ½cm/¼in.

2 Mix the berries together, then sprinkle over the yogurt along with the oats and chia seeds.

3 Cover the yogurt with another layer of kitchen foil, then place in the freezer for at least 4 hours.

4 Remove from the freezer and, using a sharp knife, carefully cut into chunks. Either place the shards in a freezer bag to use when required or allow to soften for a minute or two before giving to baby. Lasts for approximately 1 month in the freezer.

>> **MIX IT UP:**
✳ Any plant-based yogurt works well.
✳ For those over one year old, stir some honey or maple syrup into the yogurt or top with some chocolate shavings.

Ingredient
Nutritional Information

Vegetables

ASPARAGUS Vitamins A, B6, B9 (Folate), C, E, K, Calcium, Fibre, Iron, Magnesium, Potassium, Protein, Zinc

AUBERGINES/EGGPLANT Vitamins B1, B3, B6, B9 (Folate), C, K, Calcium, Copper, Fibre, Magnesium, Potassium

AVOCADOS Vitamins A, B1, B2, B3, B5, B6, B9 (Folate), C, E, K, Copper, Fibre, Iron, Magnesium, Omega-3 Fatty Acids, Potassium, Protein, Zinc

BEETROOTS/BEETS Vitamins A, B1, B2, B3, B6, B9 (folate), C, Calcium, Copper, Fibre, Iron, Magnesium, Potassium, Protein

BROCCOLI Vitamins A, B1, B2, B3, B6, B9 (Folate), C, D, E, K, Calcium, Fibre, Iron, Potassium, Protein, Zinc

BUTTERNUT SQUASH Vitamins A, B1, B3, B6, B9 (Folate), C, Calcium, Fibre, Iron, Magnesium, Potassium

CARROTS Vitamins A, C, B6, B7, B9 (Folate), K, Calcium, Fibre, Potassium

CAULIFLOWER Vitamins B6, B9 (Folate), C, K, Calcium, Fibre, Iron, Magnesium, Phosphorus, Potassium

CAVOLO NERO/BLACK KALE Vitamins A, B1, B2, B3, B6, B9 (Folate), C, K, Calcium, Copper, Iron, Fibre, Magnesium, Omega-3 Fatty Acids, Potassium, Protein

CELERY Vitamins A, B9 (Folate), C, K, Calcium, Fibre, Manganese, Potassium

CHILLIES Vitamins A, B2, B3, B6, B9 (Folate), C, E, K, Calcium, Iron, Potassium, Magnesium

COURGETTES/ZUCCHINI Vitamins A, B1, B6, B9 (Folate), C, K, Copper, Magnesium, Potassium

CUCUMBERS Vitamins A, B1, B2, B5, B6, B9 (Folate), C, K, Copper, Fibre, Magnesium, Potassium

EDAMAME Vitamins B1, B2, B9 (Folate), C, K, Calcium, Copper, Fibre, Iron, Magnesium, Potassium, Protein, Zinc

GARLIC Vitamins B1, B3, B6, B9 (Folate), C, D, E, K, Copper, Manganese, Selenium

GREEN BEANS Vitamins A, B6, B9 (Folate), C, K, Calcium, Fibre, Magnesium, Potassium

GREEN CABBAGE Vitamins A, B6, B9 (Folate), C, K, Calcium, Fibre, Iron, Magnesium, Potassium

KALE Vitamins A, B1, B2, B3, B6, B9 (Folate), C, E, K, Calcium, Copper, Fibre, Iron, Magnesium, Omega-3 Fatty Acids, Potassium, Protein

LEEKS Vitamins A, B6, B9 (Folate), C, K, Copper, Fibre, Iron, Magnesium

LETTUCE Vitamins A, B6, B9 (Folate), C, K, Fibre, Iron, Magnesium, Potassium

MUSHROOMS Vitamins B1, B2, B3, B5, B9 (Folate), C, D, Copper, Magnesium, Potassium, Selenium, Zinc

OLIVES Vitamin E, Calcium, Copper, Iron, Magnesium, Potassium

ONION/SHALLOTS Vitamins B1, B6, B7, B9 (Folate), C, E, K, Calcium, Fibre, Iron, Magnesium, Potassium

PAK CHOI/BOK CHOY Vitamins A, B6, B9 (Folate), C, K, Calcium, Fibre, Iron, Magnesium, Potassium

PEAS Vitamins A, B1, B6, B9 (Folate), C, K, Fibre, Iron, Magnesium, Potassium, Protein, Zinc

PEPPERS/BELL PEPPERS Vitamins A, B2, B3, B6, B9 (Folate), C, E, K, Fibre, Iron, Manganese, Potassium

POTATOES Vitamins B3, B6, B9 (Folate), C, Fibre, Magnesium, Potassium, Protein

ROCKET/ARUGULA Vitamins A, B9 (Folate), C, E, K, Calcium, Copper, Iron, Magnesium, Manganese, Potassium, Zinc

SAMPHIRE Vitamins A, B2, B6, B9 (Folate), B12, C, D, Calcium, Fibre, Iodine, Iron, Magnesium, Omega-3 Fatty Acids, Potassium, Zinc

SEAWEED Vitamins B2, B9 (Folate), E, K, Calcium, Copper, Fibre, Iron, Magnesium, Omega 3 Fatty Acids, Protein, Zinc

SPINACH Vitamins A, B1, B2, B6, B9 (Folate), C, E, K, Calcium, Fibre, Iron, Magnesium, Manganese, Protein, Zinc

SPRING ONIONS/SCALLIONS Vitamins A, B1, B6, B7, B9 (Folate), C, E, Calcium, Fibre, Iron, Magnesium, Potassium

SWEETCORN Vitamins B1, B3, B5, B6, B9 (Folate), C, Fibre, Magnesium, Potassium, Protein

SWEET POTATOES Vitamins A, B5, B6, B9 (Folate), C, Calcium, Copper, Fibre, Iron, Magnesium, Potassium, Zinc

TOMATOES/TOMATO PUREE/PASTE Vitamins A, B3, B5, B6, B7, B9 (Folate), C, K, Copper, Fibre, Potassium

Fruit

APPLES Vitamin A, B9 (Folate), C, E, K, Calcium, Fibre, Magnesium, Potassium

APRICOTS Vitamins A, B5, B6, C, E, Calcium, Fibre, Magnesium, Potassium

BANANAS Vitamins A, B6, B9 (Folate), C, Copper, Fibre, Iron, Magnesium, Potassium

BLUEBERRIES Vitamins A, B6, B9 (folate), C, E, K, Copper, Fibre, Magnesium

COCONUT Vitamins B6, B9 (Folate), Calcium, Copper, Iron, Potassium, Zinc

DATES Vitamins A, B3, B6, Calcium, Copper, Fibre, Iron, Magnesium, Potassium

FIGS Vitamins A, B6, K, Calcium, Fibre, Iron, Magnesium, Potassium

LEMONS Vitamins B1, B2, B6, B9 (Folate), C, Calcium, Magnesium, Potassium

LIMES Vitamins A, C, Potassium

MANGOES Vitamins B1, B2, B3, B5, B6, B9 (Folate), C, E, K, Copper, Fibre, Magnesium, Potassium

ORANGES Vitamins A, B1, B5, B9 (Folate), Calcium, Fibre, Potassium

PEARS Vitamins B9 (Folate), C, K, Copper, Fibre, Potassium

POMEGRANATES Vitamins B9 (Folate), C, E, K, Calcium, Fibre, Iron, Potassium, Protein

RAISINS Vitamins B6, C, K, Calcium, Copper, Fibre, Iron, Potassium

RASPBERRIES Vitamins A, B9 (Folate), C, E, K, Calcium, Fibre, Magnesium, Potassium

STRAWBERRIES Vitamins B6, B9 (Folate), C, E, K, Fibre, Potassium

Herbs and Spices

BASIL Vitamins A, B6, B9 (Folate), C, K, Calcium, Fibre, Iron, Magnesium

CHIVES Vitamins A, B9 (Folate), C, K

CINNAMON Vitamin K, Calcium, Fibre, Iron, Magnesium, Potassium

CORIANDER/CILANTRO Vitamins A, B9 (Folate), C, E, K, Fibre, Iron, Magnesium, Potassium

CUMIN Vitamins A, B6, C, E, K, Calcium, Copper, Iron, Magnesium, Potassium

DILL Vitamins A, C, Calcium, Iron, Magnesium

GINGER Vitamins B3, B6, B9 (Folate), C, Iron, Magnesium, Potassium, Zinc

LEMONGRASS Vitamin B9 (Folate), Calcium, Iron

MINT Vitamins A, B6, B9 (Folate), C, Calcium, Iron, Magnesium, Potassium

MUSTARD SEEDS Vitamin B1, Calcium, Iron, Magnesium, Omega-3 Fatty Acids, Protein, Zinc

OREGANO Vitamins B9 (Folate) C, E, K, Calcium, Fibre, Iron, Manganese, Potassium

PARSLEY Vitamins A, B6, B9 (Folate), C, E, K, Calcium, Fibre, Iron, Magnesium, Potassium

SAGE Vitamins A, B6, B9 (folate), K, Magnesium, Phosphorus, Potassium

THYME Vitamins A, B1, B2, B3, B5, B6, B9 (Folate), C, K, Calcium, Fibre, Iron, Magnesium, Potassium

TURMERIC Vitamins B3, B9 (folate), C, Calcium, Iron, Potassium

Dairy

BUTTER Vitamins A, B12, D, E, K, Calcium

CHEDDAR CHEESE Vitamins A, B2, B5, B6, B9 (Folate), B12, Calcium, Phosphorus, Protein, Zinc

EGGS Vitamins A, B2, B5, B6, B9 (Folate), B12, D, E, K, Calcium, Protein, Selenium, Zinc

FETA CHEESE Vitamins A, B2, B6, B9 (Folate), B12, D, K, Calcium, Phosphorus, Protein, Zinc

GREEK YOGURT Vitamins B6, B12, Calcium, Potassium, Protein, Zinc

GRUYERE CHEESE Vitamin A, B9 (Folate), B12, Calcium, Protein, Zinc

MASCARPONE CHEESE Vitamin A, Calcium, Potassium, Protein
MILK/CREAM Vitamin A, B1, B2, B3, B5, B6, B9 (Folate), B12, D, Calcium, Magnesium, Potassium, Protein, Zinc
MOZZARELLA Vitamins A, B9 (folate), Calcium, Magnesium, Potassium, Protein, Zinc
PARMESAN CHEESE Vitamins A, B12, Calcium, Cobalamin, Protein

Meat

BEEF Vitamins B6, B12, D, Iron, Magnesium, Phosphorus, Potassium, Protein, Selenium, Zinc
CHICKEN Vitamin B12, Copper, Iron, Protein, Zinc
LAMB Vitamins B3, B12, Iron, Potassium, Protein, Zinc
PORK Vitamins B1, B2, B3, B6, D, Iron, Magnesium, Potassium, Protein, Zinc

Fish

COD Vitamins A, B3, B5, B6, B12, C, E, Calcium, Magnesium, Omega-3 Fatty Acids, Potassium, Protein
HADDOCK Vitamins A, B1, B2, B3, B6, B9 (Folate), B12, D, Calcium, Magnesium, Potassium, Protein, Zinc
MACKEREL Vitamins A, B1, B2, B3, B5, B6, B12, D, E, K, Magnesium, Omega 3 Fatty-Acids, Potassium, Protein, Zinc
MONKFISH Vitamins A, B2, B3, B5, B6, B9 (Folate), B12, Calcium, Iron, Magnesium, Potassium, Protein, Zinc
PRAWNS/SHRIMP Vitamin B12, E, Calcium, Copper, Iron, Magnesium, Omega-3 Fatty Acids, Phosphorus, Potassium, Protein, Selenium, Zinc
SALMON Vitamins B1, B2, B3, B5, B6, B9 (Folate), B12, D, Magnesium, Omega-3 Fatty Acids, Potassium, Protein, Zinc
SARDINES Vitamins B3, B12, D, Calcium, Iron, Magnesium, Omega-3 Fatty Acids, Potassium, Protein, Zinc
SEA BASS Vitamin A, B1, B2, B3, B6, B12, Calcium, Iron, Magnesium, Omega-3 Fatty Acids, Zinc
TUNA Vitamins B1, B3, B6, B12, Iron, Omega 3 Fatty Acids, Magnesium, Potassium, Protein, Zinc

Pulses and Grains

ARBORIO RICE Vitamins B3, B6, Copper, Fibre, Iron, Magnesium, Protein, Zinc
BLACK RICE Vitamins B1, B2, B3, Copper, Fibre, Iron, Magnesium, Potassium, Protein, Zinc
BROWN RICE Vitamins B1, B2, B3, B6, B9 (Folate), Copper, Fibre, Iron, Magnesium, Phosphorus, Protein, Selenium, Zinc
BUCKWHEAT Copper, Fibre, Iron, Magnesium, Protein
BUTTER/LIMA BEANS B1, B2, B6, B9 (Folate), Fibre, Iron, Magnesium, Manganese, Potassium, Protein, Zinc
CANNELLINI BEANS Vitamins B2, B6, B9 (Folate), C, Calcium, Copper, Fibre, Iron, Magnesium, Potassium, Protein, Zinc
CHICKPEAS/GARBANZO BEANS Vitamins A, B1, B2, B3, B5, B6, B9 (Folate), C, Calcium, Copper, Fibre, Iron, Magnesium, Potassium, Protein, Zinc
COUSCOUS Vitamins B1, B3, B9 (Folate), Iron, Magnesium, Potassium, Protein
KIDNEY BEANS Vitamins B1, B2, B3, B5, B6, B9 (Folate), C, K, Copper, Fibre, Iron, Magnesium, Potassium, Protein
LENTILS Vitamins B1, B2, B6, B9 (Folate), Copper, Fibre, Iron, Magnesium, Protein, Zinc
OATS Vitamins B1, B3, B9 (Folate), Copper, Fibre, Iron, Magnesium, Protein, Zinc
ORZO Vitamins B1, B3, B9 (Folate), Iron, Magnesium, Protein, Zinc
SOBA NOODLES Vitamins B1, B3, Fibre, Iron, Magnesium, Potassium, Protein, Zinc
TOFU Vitamins B1, B2, B3, B6, B9 (Folate), Calcium, Copper, Iron, Magnesium, Potassium, Protein, Zinc
WHOLE-WHEAT PASTA/NOODLES/TORTILLAS/BREAD Vitamins B1, B3, B9 (Folate), Copper, Fibre, Iron, Magnesium, Protein, Zinc

Nuts and Seeds

ALMONDS Vitamins B7, B9 (Folate), E, Calcium, Fibre, Iron, Magnesium, Protein,Potassium, Riboflavin, Zinc

CASHEW NUTS Vitamins B1, B6, B9 (Folate), C, K, Copper, Fibre, Iron, Magnesium, Protein

CHIA SEEDS Calcium, Copper, Fibre, Omega-3 Fatty Acids, Potassium, Protein, Zinc

SESAME SEEDS/TAHINI Vitamins B1, B3, B6, E, Calcium, Copper, Fibre, Iron, Magnesium, Protein, Zinc

PINE NUTS Vitamins B1, B2, B3, E, Copper, Fibre, Iron, Magnesium, Manganese, Omega-3 Fatty Acids, Potassium, Protein, Zinc

PISTACHIOS Vitamins B1, B2, B3, B5, B6, B9 (folate) C, E, K, Calcium, Copper, Fibre, Magnesium, Manganese, Potassium, Protein, Selenium, Zinc

PUMPKIN SEEDS Vitamins B2, B9 (Folate), K, Calcium, Copper, Fibre, Iron, Magnesium, Omega-3 Fatty Acids, Potassium, Protein, Zinc

WALNUTS Vitamins B6, B9 (Folate), E, Copper, Fibre, Iron, Magnesium, Omega-3 Fatty Acids, Protein, Zinc

Storecupboard Ingredients

CHOCOLATE (DARK) Vitamin A, Calcium, Copper, Fibre, Iron, Magnesium, Potassium, Selenium, Zinc

COCOA POWDER Vitamins B1, B3, B5, B9, Copper, Fibre, Iron, Magnesium, Potassium, Protein, Zinc

COCONUT MILK B6, B9 (Folate), C, Calcium, Iron, Magnesium, Potassium, Protein, Zinc

COCONUT WATER Vitamin B1, B2, B3, B9 (Folate), C, Calcium, Fibre, Magnesium, Potassium

DESICCATED COCONUT Vitamins B6, B9 (Folate), Calcium, Copper, Iron, Potassium, Zinc

MAPLE SYRUP Calcium, Copper, Iron, Magnesium, Potassium, Zinc

MISO Vitamins B2, B9 (Folate), K, Calcium, Fibre, Iron, Magnesium, Potassium, Protein

PEANUT BUTTER Vitamins B3, B5, B6, B9 (Folate), E, Copper, Iron, Magnesium, Potassium, Protein, Zinc

POLENTA/CORNMEAL Vitamins A, C, Fibre, Iron, Magnesium, Protein, Zinc

Index

21982320263761